I'VE ONLY GOT ONE...

...But Its a Beauty!!

Kean Turner

authorHOUSE®

AuthorHouse™ UK Ltd.
500 Avebury Boulevard
Central Milton Keynes, MK9 2BE
www.authorhouse.co.uk
Phone: 08001974150

First published by AuthorHouse   06/16/2011

ISBN: 978-1-4567-7187-4

Cancer is not a laughing matter........but laughter does matter.

Laugh at yourself

Your imagination is a beautiful gift, use it like children do and watch its magic weave miracles in your world.

Kean Turner

The hurt it hit like a dog down a pit
With the scent of a rabbits mane
The sun it shone but the bright had gone
Like acid in a summer rain
The pain it eased and grinded
Then stalled like a cart with a blistered wheel
Flesh fled......... worrying,
Kissing her soul goodbye
How the dawn it broke and the light it spoke
As the soul then felt alive
For bliss came running, like tears that rolled
For the brightest star was born.

Kean Turner

The wise write that there is not a shred of evidence in support of the idea that life is meant to be serious.

Life is far too important for that.

Do the stars that dance in your children's eyes, tell you that they would rather frown than laugh?

ACKNOWLEDGEMENTS

Thank you to Linda for typing up my first draft of scribbled nonsense, you set me on my way.

Where do I start with Fiona….? for proof reading and making valuable suggestions and for being a true friend.

Thank you to Craig Fee for your photography and ideas.

Thank you to Fanny, you know who you are!

I offer my eternal gratitude to the doctors and nurses who continue to work tirelessly in demanding times, especially my friend Helen

For my dear friend Bill who continues to shine in my heart, we all miss you Boo.

Thank you for our boy….CLC

Thank you, Paul Birchall for telling the world about this book.

To my left testicle, without you, there could be no book.

Contents

Chapter 1

1972 - I am a Boy

At six years old I remember hearing my dad tell a man I was born the year England won the world cup, in 1966. I didn't know how long it would be until they told me that I was seven, I don't think I cared and I certainly didn't worry. Frowning and looking sad was for the big people.

Worrying was alien to me and the other kids that were part of my life. My only concerns back then were having enough time for skipping, belly aching laughter, sniggering at poops, picking fights with invisible enemies, having fun and poking earwigs out of holes in garden posts with lolly sticks. I would swing on the gate, passing the time of day, dreaming of being a soldier.

Winning that world cup for England made me feel special. It was as if I had scored the winning goals myself. Dad seemed happy as he brought it up in conversation with people he met who asked how old his daughter was. Yes I looked like a girl, with big eyes, a gentle complexion and long fair hair. If Twiggy needed a body double, I was

1

the one. If winning world cups made dad and everyone else happy, then I was all for winning cups. I liked to be happy and it felt good when others were too. Thank you Mr Bobby Moore and thank you to me, for what ever it was I did that made all the grown ups happy and smile about the time I was born.

Oh yes.......and thank you to mum and dad for that holiday in Skegness in 1965 and your 3 minutes of pleasure that resulted in the boy that looked like a girl that wrote these words.

Dad must have kept that cup in a cupboard somewhere; one of those cupboards that no one goes in, I never did get to see it in the house.

Mum had a fine pair of lungs for a small pretty woman, she would scream at me as I looked around the house for the "Jules Rimet" cup*" forget that bloody cup and come and eat your tea"*.

My life was about having fun, sticking fingers in grandmas chocolate cake, running after pigeons while out with grandad and laughing at the top of my voice as he fights for breath after another Capstan full cigarette.

He must have loved chasing me around the market, panting like a porn star with asthma and sweating like a cow off to slaughter. Finally I would be caught and the toy shop routine would begin, bribing me to behave with the lure of a bright coloured plastic hammer or a box of toy soldiers. It always worked and I was soon back under the control of one of the serious people.

It's easy to forget now as an adult just how big everything seemed back then. The grown ups seemed like giants and their words seemed longer and complicated. As a child it was the simple things that appealed. Who needed complications? There was no room in my life for trauma and upset, if it came along I didn't welcome it, I would rather have one of the big people deal with it. Mum could look after my cuts and bruises and fill my stomach up with food. Dad could look after the football side and kick a ball about with me and my older brother in the square outside our house.

Dad could continue working at the sweet factory forever. I loved the smell of him when he came in at night, mint, sweet and sugary, now and again his white work cap would hit me full on in the face and the smell of the factory filled my lungs. It was a calming inviting aroma. I asked countless questions, I didn't really absorb the answers and was frequently told to be quiet. Although the house was full of sweets and the cupboards bursting at the seams from dad bringing home the broken chocolates, there could never be enough for me. I was relentless for more, wherever we went I would ask mum for this and for that. *"I should have called you, can I have"*, she would say as I pestered her for something new, anything would do. My favourite and best of all was the lucky bag. It felt like a suitcase of fun, an oasis of surprise. A great big bright green paper bag with a big purple dragon on the front, adorned with bright letters inviting my enquiring mind to dive in and drown myself in the junk inside.

In tender moments mum would bend down in front of me ,look right into my eyes and tell me I had big brown beady eyes, I didn't know what beady meant, but I knew it made me feel good , just by the way she said the words. She would run the side of her finger down my cheek and gently touch the tip of my nose; making me blink ....I knew mum loved me.

Chapter 2

BIG BRO

My brother on the other hand, didn't seem to like me, if he did; he certainly struggled to show it. How different we were. He was so much older than me, when I was six he was nine, when I was seven he was ten. Why couldn't I catch him up? I could never get my head around it. He loved being older and so much bigger and stronger. I was confused that if my so called big brother loved me as much as mum says, then why does he hold me down and fart on me at every opportunity. How come he only does it when mum and dad are out of the way? I would hold my breath for what seemed forever until the stench and his big fat arse had left the building. My young mind was tortured and confused. How was it that I could cope and enjoy my own farts and even love the way they smelt and lingered? But loathe my brothers. It was very confusing. We did after all eat pretty much the same food.

If he wasn't tossing me across the bed, holding me down and letting rip, he would be teasing and giving me dead legs, a sharp dig to the thigh that stopped me in my tracks. Life at times was about avoiding people who wanted to fart, tickle or kiss me. The girl next door was one I did my best to avoid, at 12years old she was more like one of the big people, although she didn't have balloons down her top the size of mums, she was still bigger and stronger than me. She had a fascination with drenching me in her spit and hugging me as hard as she could. She was obsessed with squeezing the life out of me. Thankfully my worst nightmare never did materialize, being cornered by them both ,her soaking my face with spit while my brother roles the crack of his arse across my face and letting rip for England. The two of them kept me on my young toes.

At times I was allowed to play out on my own; although it was never far from home. I would play with anyone that seemed to be the same size as me. I avoided the bigger kids and wet lips from next door and felt much safer with kids who like me, didn't wish to wet, hurt, fart or fight.

Chapter 3

COCK

Cock was a pal of mine; I can't remember his real name. He became a friend along with some other kids the same age, the first time I met him I was kicking a ball against a wall. I was in my own world pretending to be George Best.

As I blasted the ball against the wall and strained my voice creating the sound of a barmy Old Trafford crowd, I felt a presence nearby. I turned my head around and not two feet away stood a boy the same size as me. He didn't speak, he just stood staring. He had a face as serious as granddads when he realised that he had no cigs left and the shops were shut. Cock looked right into my face. I stared back; it was like a scene from the black and white cowboy film I had watched that morning.

He stood with one hand on his hip, like a modern day Jessie James, his other hand, pulling down with great determination the waistband on his dark brown cotton slacks. His penis and balls were hanging out like washing on a line and his stare and manner invited me to look at his package of love. I picked up my ball and stared full on. With my football under my arm I was mesmerised by his package. It was the surprise of his introduction and not the chicken fillet that hung in the morning sun that intrigued me. What a greeting! His stare seemed to last forever. His harvest festival reminded me of the green balloon that hung in the top corner of our living room that had been there since before Christmas.

Neither of us said a word. We were like two gun slingers, the weapon he drew might not have been loaded, but it did look dangerous.

What did this kid want? What did he want me to do? Aim mine at his? Is this a duel? Then what? Will he pee on me? Will I pee on him? But I didn't want a pee. I had never met anyone in this manner before; I wasn't sure what was expected. I knew I had a cricket bat close by, should I crack him? Should I crack it? After all it did seem longer than the one I had. Somehow I knew we wouldn't be mates if I did. I felt awkward but at the same time, curious. Do all kids attract this kind of attention? I bounced my ball and decided against returning the favour. I kept my tackle in its holster. There was a silence in the air......an air of anticipation and then loud laughter. My laughter was more relief as he carefully slipped it back into his cotton slacks.

Thankfully there was no trace of urine from either of us. As we played slam together I kept one eye on him. This kid needed watching. Some older kids nicknamed him Cock. I had realised why. The name stuck for the rest of his childhood. Whenever he met anyone for the first time, out it came, it didn't matter who it was. Passing cars, full buses, adults, kids, they all got the same treatment. Cock was not bothered in the slightest, he loved it... The only person he didn't greet in this fashion was his dad.

After a while we stopped laughing at him, but he always persisted. It was as if he was addicted to the sound of people's laughter and the importance and acceptance that it gave him. We didn't care though, he was our friend. He was a one off.

It was awkward at times having a mate with a strange name. One day we called for him and asked his dad to see if he minded getting his little cock out........... He wasn't amused. His dad was scary, a giant of a man with stubble and a filthy white vest with stains and a permanent cigarette stuck to his lip. He looked us up and down, his mouth carrying a reminder of his dinner in either corner. He didn't look happy. Our innocence had dropped Cock right in it. As the big red door slammed in our faces the power of his words bellowed through their house. *"Margaret, he's had it out again".* Banging and shouting then followed as we made tracks down the path. He didn't allow anyone to play with his little Cock for a few days, soon enough though, out little Cock came, balls and all. There were advantages for Cock; no one ever took a sweet off him, unless it was in a wrapper.

He was an endearing little Cock and he taught me something wonderful.

Something that I have tried to carry with me throughout my life.....no I don't mean getting my genitalia out at the drop of a hat......let me explain.

One evening I was sat at home and I tried to pronounce the word hippopotamus. I struggled with the awkward word and couldn't get my tongue around it, my mother laughed out loud at my attempt. I tried again and again and the word just would not come. Mum carried on laughing; she eventually cupped my cheeks in her hand and blessed me for trying. Thereafter I deliberately messed with words; in the hope I might again hear the sound of laughter being directed at me. I felt the immediate warmth that Cock must have received the first time someone laughed at him. I had learned a wonderful gimmick. I realised why Cock, got his cock out. I had felt how he felt, that first time he'd heard and felt the warmth of laughter created by his actions, I felt special, for I had done this with a word, an awkward clumsy word at that. I had no need to flash my privates at anyone to get my fix. But I knew there and then why Cock did it and felt as though I understood him a little more. It would be a path I would try to keep on, getting by with laughter as my friend. Cock could keep getting his cock out if it made him feel better, but that was not for me. There would be plenty of times in the future for people to look at my genitalia when rather I wish they wouldn't. The sound of laughter was great to my young ears. It made me feel wanted; it made me feel loved and it made me feel special. I soon worked out that if someone was laughing at you, there was a good chance they couldn't hurt you. Would laughter stop wet lips next door? Or would it encourage her to pounce? I decided not to try Cocks trick on her, it might backfire and maybe she would want me even more and we might even end up getting married. I avoided her as much as I could. It was funny because she never went anywhere near Cock, she'd just scream when he came anywhere near.

Chapter 4

WHEN I WASN'T PLAYING WITH MY ANGRY NEIGHBOUR'S COCK

Most days were spent getting up early, raiding the sweet cupboard. Leaving as little trace of me as possible near the bags of broken chocolate and toffee crisps that dad brought home from the sweet factory where he worked. I wished he would work there forever.

I would pretend to shoot all the neighbours windows out with my imaginary rifle. Hoping that wet lips would pop her head through the curtains and I could blast her and send her big fat wet sloppy lips to kingdom come.

I would dream of one day being as big and as strong as her and holding her down and sharing my earwigs. I would grab a clump of grass from our overgrown garden and throw it towards her house, as if it was a grenade. Making the sound of an explosion, pouting my lips as the saliva flew out in the direction of her bedroom. She and my brother were the enemy. How I wished to have my brother's gift of being able to fart at will. He just seemed to be a never ending stinking fart machine. How did he

10

do it? I was baffled. He had an amazing gift, but why must he practice this on me. He takes great delight in releasing this gift on me, and then spends hours laughing as I struggle to escape the stench. I prayed mum would get me a younger brother for me to fart on. It got to the point where I would no longer resist and just waited my lips as tight as his buttocks.

Between hating and hiding from Bonnie and Clyde I would sit in the garden daydreaming. As I broke the stems off dandelions, I'd wonder if this is what they made dandelion and burdock from and what exactly was burdock.

I would draw on the path with the head of the flower until the yellow ran out. Looking into the middle of the broken stem and running my fingers down the white wet substance then toss it aside into the long grass. Quickly getting bored I'd then look into the cloudy blue sky and look for patterns in the clouds, like how dad had shown me . I would see something, a horse, a face and just as quickly it would be gone. I only had thoughts for there and then and it seemed that there could only ever be now. There was no need to worry about tomorrow or yesterday. The only time I wished for tomorrow was if I had been told we were doing something exciting. Or if wet lips next door was up against a firing squad for scaring the kids with her big round rubber sucking lips. I would stand up and kick the tips of the long grass and set free the 1 o'clock 2 o'clock plants that lived side by side with the dandelions. I never knew their real names, just that mum had told me they were there for telling the time to the fairies. I would snap the heads off and blow and count to as many as I could. I would set free all the soft seeds and watch them dance in the air. I would pull at them with my fingers and watch them glide away on the wind.

On summer days I would fly in the house at the sound of the ice cream mans bell, ringing out on our street. Begging mum for a Screwball Special (a plastic cone filled with ice-cream with a bubbly hidden in the bottom) with bright red juice resting like mountain snow and a plastic spoon to devour it with. I was in heaven. Not every attempt with mum was a success though, *"no it will ruin your tea"* came her reply. I would then screw my face up in the world's worst sulking session.

Sulking should have then been made an Olympic event I would have walked away with the gold medal. I remember seeing my dear old gran of 90 and thinking boy could that old girl sulk!! She never had any teeth in and I would be amazed at how she always seemed so heartbroken. With all the money in her purse, she would be able to buy the biggest ice-cream in the world and still she looks like she's trying to eat herself.

As the van sets off to the next street, the realisation that I'm not going to get one today would kick in and my whole body would tense up in anger and injustice. The sulking never lasted, it wasn't allowed to, because although mum was fare she was firm and if my dad thought I had been a bad lad whilst he was at work I would be for it.

At times I was lucky, as the music of the bell worked its magic down the street I would be again at mum's heels begging for a cone. *"You can still catch it mum if you hurry"*. She would give me a look grab her purse, throw the tea towel on the side and then go in the cupboard and bring out a glass trifle dish. The pride I felt heading for the van with mum at my side knowing that the man was going to fill the dish up and it's all coming back to our house, was magical. I would look at the other kids watching the van who I knew hadn't been as lucky as me and feel so very special. My mum, this lady here with the big boobie doobies and dish and red purse is treating us to heaven. On the way back the paper napkin would be bursting with wafers. I was one happy kid. I had a wonderful feeling of pride and although I didn't understand the word, I knew the feeling. This was my mum and my mum comes to the ice cream van with me.

The trifle dish would then collect dust at the back of the cupboard until our next ice-cream treat, it would eventually become the home of the resident goldfish. When the rains came and my nose stuck to the cold window, praying for the chance to play outside, Cliff Richard's "Congratulations" rang through the house as mum blasted the furniture with her magic duster, skipping and dancing around the furniture and spinning and pulling my cheek as she went. I loved it when mum looked happy; strangely it was usually when Dad was at work. Cliff would eventually drone off into my boredom and she'd try and liven it up for me by sticking Pinkie and Perky on the record deck.

The orange disks floated magically if not smoothly around the turntable and mum thought I was in heaven. The high pitched voices of the piglets went through me after a while and I was soon bored and looking for something else to do.

When dad was in the house I had to behave, we never knew what kind of mood he was in. His voice was loud and when dad and mum shouted at each other I prayed for Pinkie and Perky's return. The shouting and banging about was happening more and more. Playing out was my escape. If the weather was bad, then going to my room with my imagination for company was always a good option. I would sit and talk to myself on the bed, my own company was better than listening to mum and dad shouting at each other. I would start to put the world right....why has my brother an obsession with farting? He was so lucky to have a smaller thinner attractive brother and if I had one, I would cherish him, cuddle him, and give him my toys, share things with him, teach him , read to him, stroke him until he slept, then bray him with a plastic hammer. Maybe when I'm nine or ten I would hold him down and explain to him why I am about to fart on him. I would educate him and get him used to the stench that comes from another kids arse.

When it becomes silent downstairs I creep out of my room and slide down the stairs, bumping down every step from top to bottom. Sliding down the carpet, I'd dislodge half a dozen bright green plastic 1970,s gripper rods. Dad had either stormed out or been thrown out, it's usually one or the other. All I am bothered about is the quiet that the house now holds. Creeping off the bottom step I hear mum crying and I open the door to her....I hate it when she cries. I take any chance I can to steal a cuddle and its always a good time after they've been shouting and screaming as mum's arms are usually wide open for me. She'd say *"You've got big beady eyes"*, what ever they are, but it feels good, again as she says the words, she looks right into my eyes and I know she's being kind, just by the sound of her voice. I want to help her but I can't, so I just accept my cuddle and try and make her smile. I ask if she is friends with dad and I'm always told that there is nothing to worry about. Mum always puts it right. If I bang my leg, fall off the gate and bang my head, it's not long before the Dettol comes out, it stinks, but I trust her. It reminds my young mind of the doctors and old women, and mum makes out it will mend my grazes and knocks.

Chapter 5

A DROP OF THE HARD STUFF

It's the same with Indian Brandy whenever I fain illness or stomach ache, out it comes, she waters it down with warm water out of the kettle and I'm made to down it, it usually takes 349 sips to sink it. It drops into my stomach like a stone thrown in a well. I explode inside and shout for assistance from the child police, this woman should be locked up. The fire water is 70% proof and I'm drunk for the rest of the day.

Within minutes I'm leering at the neighbours through the letter box, shouting abuse. Poor old Mrs Yates a lovely 78 year old grandma of 5 is passing our house. When sober I have a lot of time for her, as she is always really kind to me. In my Indian Brandy state all this goes out of the window, *"YOU GREY HAIRED OLD WITCH"* I scream. She stands at the foot of the garden in disbelief staring at the door, her eyes focusing on the letterbox. After looking around to see if anyone is watching, she sticks up her index finger on her left hand and raises it to the sky. She mutters something in retaliation under her breathe and storms off. Another sip of the hard stuff and my stomach ache has gone; my insides feel like Tenerife in August! No wonder dad likes a pint. I drop mum's keys in the trifle dish, nearly knocking the fish unconscious…. I'm plastered, I take a liking to it and wrestle the bottle out of her hand and were grappling on the floor.

I escape her grip and return to the letter box. Next up it's the postman's turn. He's trying to force a letter into my mouth through the gap and is startled. He steps backward away from the high pitched tripe coming out of my mouth. *"GET OUT OF OUR GARDEN AND TAKE YOUR SACK WITH YOU!"*. He defends himself with a word I hadn't come across before, *"T**T"*. I'm the worlds youngest drunk and I've convinced myself I'm indestructible. Poor mum is startled, shattered, watching in disbelief. The brandy soon wears off and although my stomach no longer aches my head does. I'm then carried up to bed and left to sleep it off, while poor mum ponders what to do with the crowd of people in the garden upset by my outbursts. The postman is on the verge of resignation; Mrs Yates has come back and is white with rage and threatening legal action, she then starts on the postman about one of her missing parcels. Mum is dismayed and finishes off the brandy and flirts with the post man. Another neighbour complains about the *"Get your penis out"* chants aimed at him as he returned home from work. Mum explained it wasn't her and that she is trying her best to be happily married; he leaves the scene disappointed and puts his penis back in his trousers.

I slept my Indian Brandy hangover off and woke up next morning, oblivious to the havoc I'd caused.

Chapter 6

I'LL CALL HIM, BRIAN

My next strange encounter occurred when mum allowed me to stay at one of her friend's house for tea; I lapped up the opportunity to be free spending time playing with someone else's toys. I hardly knew the boy and was to stay the afternoon with him at his house, I think my mum knew his mum, a kind of mutual agreement to give them some much needed peace.

On arrival at the house mum dropped me off, gently kissed my cheek and set off down the path, reassuring me that she would pick me up in a few hours. For legal reasons I'll call this boy Brian. On entering his play room, Brian took it on himself to turn into Big Daddy, the famous wrestler of the time. *"Do you want a wrestle?.* I politely declined his offer. Too late......!He hadn't waited for my answer and within seconds my leg was up my back, my arm round the back of my head and my fingers were being bent in the opposite direction with which God intended. I lay on his bunk with his knee across my neck and my head hanging over the edge of his bed. *"Submit...Submit"* he wailed.........Submit? What is this maniac on about? I could not reply as my tongue was being forced into my cheek through clenched teeth. As he demanded I submit, I lay there, my eyes forced to stare in the direction of the skirting board, silently praying for some strength or for mum to come and rescue me. By now he was bouncing on my back with all his weight with my head sandwiched between his knee and arm. On my release, I lay on the bed and was then cracked across the head with a tin tray, the one that had previously held our pop and crisps. On about the 8th bang of the tray, I flipped. Bollocks to my manners I thought, bollocks to wanting his mum to say to my mum what an adorable child I was and bollocks to this lunatic. I dragged the tray out of his hand, threw him onto the bed and began returning the compliment.

His head, his back and any part of him that happened to be in the way, got it. He lay there sobbing, holding his head, wailing for me to stop. On the last crash of the tray I felt a presence in the room and low and behold watching her lovely wrestling son getting a pasting was his mum. The look of disgust on her face haunts me to this day. What was this boy that looks like a girl doing to her beautiful son? I began to feel like a victim as she pointed her long finger inches from my face with a look that resembled my grandad straining on the loo. I felt the telling off I got was very harsh, considering my twenty minutes of torture at the hands of her delightful boy. I ate my fish fingers and chips in total silence as she glared at me throughout the meal. After tea she told us to go and play in the garden and instructed me not to pick on Brian again and said that there were names for people like me. I looked at her in wonder and said *"Kean Turner."*

On entering the garden I saw another side to Brian, if I thought the wrestling was odd, the next thing he said to me, really set the alarm bells ringing! *"Come on; let's watch our Sarah have a shit behind the garage".* Sarah was his younger sister. I must have had an ear infection I remember thinking, as I am sure he has just asked me to watch his sister have a shit. No.... my ears were fine, he was serious. Before I could summon a grown up to report him to, he was off, clambering through bushes at the back of the garden and in to a clearing behind his garage.

Sarah was already there and waiting for her audience. Was this really happening? *"Ready when you are Sarah",* came Brian's encouraging words.

As she crouched down resembling a weight lifter ready to lift the bar and with Brian egging her on, I realised that my family although not entirely normal, were not remotely in the same league as this bunch. Sarah's concentration was to be admired, she stared ahead and I was transfixed with her facial expressions. She was trying with all her might to deliver for her audience. *"Go on Sarah.....Push... Push"* yelled Brian. I remember thinking what he must be like on Christmas day morning when he gets something that he really liked. Eventually she produced for Brian, she had delivered his prize, and Sarah stood up, straightened her clothing and vanished into the bushes, she seemed pleased with her afternoons work.

As I stood next to Brian, he looked into my eyes for a reaction; I stood there mesmerised by what I had just witnessed. *"What about that little beauty?",* he piped up, as he prodded it with a stick. He crouched down and stared into it.

It crossed my mind to offer him the pile I had in my underpants that had arrived when his mum was pointing her finger in my face.

I suddenly had a great urge to go home and never to return. Mum came to collect me and on the way home asked what we had been doing. All her questions were greeted with silence, all evening I sat there staring into space. I heard her ask dad what they may have given me to eat as I looked vacant and in need of sunlight. I knew that if I told her I had bent a tray onto Brian's head, been told off by his mum and watched the delightful Sarah shit for England behind the garage, she'd take me straight to see a doctor.... I chose to remain silent.

I slept that evening like never before, I dreamt about the garage, the wrestle, the pile of shit and Sarah. On waking up I wondered why there wasn't any toilet roll hanging up behind the garage? How many times had Sarah done that? And why does Sarah do that there in the first place? And how come her brother's involved? I didn't have the answers, so I put it down to one of life's little mysteries.

Chapter 7

MARTIANS AT GRAN & GRANDAD'S HOUSE

There were always new things to learn being a kid. Like the realisation that ginger nut biscuits have to be dunked in coffee just so you could swallow them. With this realisation came the confusion that I was then being told off by grandad for doing just that. How on earth was I supposed to eat these things without making them a bit softer and how come grandad eats them with ease when his teeth are nocturnal. When I stay at their house his teeth stare at me through a glass while he sleeps, I wondered why mine weren't able to pop out at will.

Life loved to confuse me. Boy was I mixed up. On waking up at their house and visiting the bathroom in the morning after I had pissed all over the wall and toilet seat, I left the room. I was to be greeted by gran walking across the landing, but what had happened to her face? When she put me to bed last night she looked normal. Her eyes were the same, but her mouth was as saggy as one of my socks. When she spoke, she spat. Her mouth was like a jelly. Her words didn't have endings. She glided past me into the bathroom as if in a trance. I stood outside the bathroom waiting. Had I been sleep walking? Had I woken up in a toothless world? I checked with my tongue and thankfully I still had my teeth. I peeped through the crack in their bedroom door and granddad was grunting with his eyes closed while his teeth looked on.

At the other side of the bed was the other matching set, they must be grandma's teeth? My God! I didn't even know. What was it about adults? Why do they do this? As she came out of the bathroom I received the first telling off of the day. I grasped the odd word as she spit at me with her loose lips. Was this really my gran? I just didn't understand it. It didn't look or sound like the woman that tucked me up in bed the night before. It was as if I had two sets of grand parents, all living in the same house.

It started to talk again, *"Cernt yoo cerntrool yer sellf werrn yooooov ad aa wee, yerv peesed all ova the waaallll."* Is there a translator in the house? This thing that had taken over my grandma's body then had the cheek to get in her bed, sit up, and try to communicate with me. It started with a sort of smile; this thing also looked like that party balloon that had slowly deflated and hung lifeless in the corner of the room, 10 days after Christmas. I was transfixed watching it try to speak. The thing even smoked. I watched as it lifted a cigarette to its rubber jaw and tossed the cigarette in. It moved the cigarette about, from one end of its mouth to the other like a caterpillar munching lettuce. Eventually the cigarette was clamped in what resembled our pet dogs bum hole. It struck a match and lit the cig, when it took its first drag; I thought it was going to turn itself inside out. All its face seemed to be pulled from within. Eventually it blew the smoke out toward me like a set of 16th Century bellows. The process was repeated until the room was filled with smoke and the other toothless wonder lying next to her started to move. It grunted, sat up and repeated the process. What a sight greeted my young eyes, my two heroes, sitting up together in bed, trying to talk to me in their best slurs. Their cigarettes danced in time as I was lovingly smoked upon.

And as If by magic, I got my family back, simultaneously they slipped their teeth in after shaking, then drying them on the duvet. The life came back into their faces as the glasses emptied and their heads filled. I was mesmerised by the transformation.

I loved all of them! I never did see all four of them together in one room. In time I grew to understand the strange language of the two rubber faced smoke suckers, strangely enough they only surfaced first thing in the morning or very late at night. The next day back at home I didn't tell mum about the four of them living at gran's house as she seemed to have enough going on arguing with dad. The following morning, as I fought the sleep that clung to my eyelashes, I urinated with ease over our own toilet seat, wall, towels and bathmat. It was a kind of calling card. I knew dad loved it when his bum met my urine on the seat first thing in the morning. I was uninterested in what was in my way for my first wee of the day. Why should I be bothered, it was great being a kid. It seemed to me, that it was the adults who made life difficult. I decided to try my luck for a cuddle and went to mum and dads room to jump in their bed. My world came crashing down, for sitting up in the same pose as gran and granddad were another two smoke suckers resembling mum and dad. They too had been taken over by the slurring, sunken faced, deflated balloon smoking creatures. It was just like back at grandmas' house, two

23

sets of teeth sat at either side of the bed. Dad's face was sunk, mum's face was sunk, and both spoke like drunks as they bellowed their smoke toward me. Sod the cuddle I'll go and get a toffee crisp. As I munched on my first chocolate bar of the day I thought about how my whole family had turned into Dr Who monsters. It was bad enough hearing the theme tune on the TV as I hid behind the sofa, but now the strange creatures were living not only at Grans but also at our house.

Chapter 8

MY OWN WORLD...WHERE IT'S SAFE

Mum and dad in between swapping teeth only seemed to want to shout at each other. I went deeper and deeper into my own world. I was in a world where nothing mattered only having fun and laughing. I would talk to myself and get lost in my imagination. It was clear that things were not right as the house was full of tension, maybe they had mixed their teeth up. Why couldn't they just swap them back and give each other a cuddle .It wasn't as simple as that though. Mum and dad had problems. I shut it out best I could. I knew things were not right. My brother sat with me one day and put his arm around me. This was serious, he didn't fart once, and if he was being nice then something was definitely wrong.

Things were happening in the household. It was even having a major affect on Duke our Jack Russell dog. He took to listening to Tony Blackburn on the radiogram with earphones which he acquired to escape the tension. Whistling away he'd sit in the corner, sipping cognac with a bowl of nibbles on his lap. It eventually got so bad Duke started eating its own muck to get itself out of a telling off for shitting in the house. I thought, hang on a minute I'm not going down that path. I get a bollocking for my bathroom antics, there's no way I'm going to lick the piss off the seat as well. I decided to teach Duke where the cloths were kept, the cleaning fluid and the dustpan and brush so he could clean it up before mum and dad found it. No wonder his breath stunk. He'd wink at me, as he licked dad's face, I would stare in wonder as dad kissed and stroked him and got his tongue involved like my big brother eating a toffee apple. Duke really took to cleaning and would eventually own his own cleaning business in Harrogate. He employed 23 people until he sold up and moved to Monaco for tax reasons with Barbara, a show poodle who he met on a speed dating evening in Battersea.

I was constantly getting told off by all the grown ups. In my family it was a case of children should be seen and clearly not heard. It felt that if you were young and small you were insignificant. I was always been talked over and not listened to. These grown ups were a pain in the backside. It was ok when they were all laughing at my antics, but as soon as I had anything serious to say, it didn't seem to register. Every child I knew had a glint in their eye, our eyes seemed to shine, and strangely enough none of the adults around me seemed to have that sparkle. They all seemed so serious. Surely they weren't born that way. I decided I wanted to stay my size and remain happy and care free forever. Who says they have all the answers? How come they fall out with each other all the time and never seem to make up. I would go through best friends like gran went through Benson and Hedges and still end up happy. Kids didn't know what a grudge was and never had enough time to hold onto one in the first place. Mum and Dad were at each other more and more and the silence never seemed to last long. I started to block out the shouting but had a fairly good idea from the bits that I had picked up that my family was on the verge of big changes.

One day after school something serious happened. Dad's at work and mum with her 2 boys in tow, leave a cosy warm home with central heating and wall to wall carpeting, to move up into Bradshaw which was really high up like a big mountain but later found out it wasn't a mountain at all, just a hill!. We arrive at a cottage on Bradshaw Rowe. There are half a dozen of these cottages all in a line, the alarm bells should have been ringing for mum straight away. Only one was occupied. The others stood, mimicking Berlin streets of 1945. I wanted to go home; I clung to mum's hand and hoped it was all a big mistake and we were here, just visiting this old lady before the whole building was demolished. How wrong I was. I would have volunteered to press the detonator and we could drop the old dear off at the bus stop at the bottom of the hill. Whatever had happened to mum to bring us here? I may have only been a young boy, but I could tell that mum was not happy. My brother's screwed up face and staring eyes along with the smell of damp was not filling my little heart with joy.

Bradshaw Rowe was up a mud track in the centre of Bradshaw village, a lovely sleeping community, with farmhouses, rolling hills and views over Halifax to die for. It was a beautiful setting, ideal for ramblers and walkers and people wanting the peace of the country side. On another occasion I would have jumped at the chance of staying, but all I wanted was home, the home I knew and more than anything my dad. Mum informed us that this was now our home, any questions directed at her about going back to live with dad, were quickly silenced.

It was a picture postcard location, perched high up on the hillside, but boy was it damp. It was idyllic and the scenery was beautiful, but our cottage at top of the hill was in need of repair. Mum must surely have known what a dump it was and she must have been really unhappy to bring her two boys to a place like this. The old lady next door, gave mum the key and she opened the door. There was a photo of a family of goats discarded on the mantelpiece that had only just left. The creaking door woke the barn owl, who in turn woke the bats, who in turn woke the rats, who then told the mice that they had better scarper as the new tenants had arrived. Was this where the story of the three bears was written? I peered around the door. We all stood there looking in. There were more animals in there than Chester Zoo! A newspaper on the floor was dated 1066; the headline stated *"Harold had taken one in the eye"*. I looked at the sports page on the back and was instructed to buy a copy in 800 years, as football hadn't been invented yet. Mum walked in first, she trod carefully, like they do in the movies when they think their in a mine field. We both followed, and then the old lady was next. She piped up *"It just needs a lick of paint and the fire lighting and it will be just like home"*. I was curious; I had never met a woman with a beard before. She had hairs coming out of the top of her nose. The mole on her face resembled a welcome mat with short hard hairs sitting perfectly in line. I was tempted to wipe by boots on it. Grey hairs pierced the air from her ears and resembled the sparklers; I soon hoped I would wave as we watched this place burn. She walked with a stoop and looked as if she was on the verge of falling apart. Her beard scared me and her thick woollen jumper hung over her thin frame. Her cat followed us in and she introduced it as Barney. *"You'll need a cat as you get a lot of field mice here"* she said. What kind of field mice occupies houses I remembered thinking. Shouldn't they change their names to "squatters." She let mum know she would sort us a cat out to help with the mice and set off on her tour. Mum was being positive, saying things like *"this is our new home, were going to have loads of fun living here"*. My brother's face was a picture; you could tell he hated it. He muttered under his breathe his disapproval. I asked him what he meant by a shit hole? I got one of those looks that I was now getting used to.

I watched the Owl pack up his belonging and set off with his suitcase under his wing. There was cracked paint hanging off the walls and the smell of damp was as prominent as the mouse shit. There was an open fire and only one room downstairs to live in. A tiny staircase led us upstairs to two small bedrooms; the floor creaked heavily as we looked in. The smell of damp was worse up stairs and the walls were wet through, paper hung off the walls like delicate leaves in autumn. If I hadn't been full of adventure I would have hated it. I knew my brother didn't like it and sensed mum felt the same, but at least the shouting had stopped between mum and dad. Even though I did miss him, mum did her best to make it feel like home. It was so damp and cold that we all had to live in the downstairs room. I knew this was serious and would keep asking when we could go back home and see dad.

There was a barbaric looking outside toilet across the cracked and broken flags outside the cottage. It had a perfect circle in the middle of the wood that reminded me of the the donkey derby at Skegness. I thought of dad getting excited as he tried to win a token for a prize, in happier times. I knew though there wouldn't be anything worth winning in here. Newspaper, replaced soft toilet roll that had been torn lovingly into small squares by the old woman. It was placed in a pile behind the seat and the cobwebs against the whitewashed walls were not at all inviting. I wasn't scared of spiders at that age, but I was wary of the dark corners and where they might creep. I would constantly be on guard. I would wait and wait until I was nearly bursting, praying I didn't have to go in there on my own. This was the early 1970's and not the turn of the century, but it was a different world away from the comforts of my old home. There were some things in life that I strangely enjoyed as a child. My bathroom experience was one of them, but sadly it was being ruined by the eyes of staring spiders. I didn't enjoy the bitter cold wind that came under the door and the cold hard newspaper that met my backside. It was the same feeling I got at school when salad was on the menu. I would hold my trousers up as far as I could, not wanting to touch the floor, to avoid unwanted visitors. I would try and keep my bum off the cold grey rough wood. The strain on my legs was unbearable, as I balanced on my toes, with one hand gripping my pants and the other between the hard seat and my bottom, so as not to touch anything that didn't belong to me. All the time my other eye was on the spider in the corner, why did they choose to live in here, and I would silently shout "please, *please stop staring at me"*. Balancing at my best, I would wipe my bum in one swipe and fly through the door, shivering, hoping nothing had landed or crawled into my trousers. I would shake my pants and pray I wouldn't need to go again in the night. I would cross examine mum, *"why can't I go to the toilet in the house where we left dad and why can't I flush it?"* This must have got mum thinking and the poor girl clearly wasn't relishing emptying it . At the end of our first week, mum decided we had to help empty the toilet. She chose a farmer's wall, as far away from grey beard as possible. Off we went. The bucket swished in her hand as we followed behind. We had been instructed to follow her to the edge of a field. Her neck did its best impression of a tortoise as she strained and pulled away with her head against the weight of the load. She walked, held her breath, stopped, breathed out in a gust and walked and strained again. She looked to be in agony as she pulled her body as tight as she could away from the stench. There must have been a good five day's worth and we followed behind like two chicks following mother duck to the river. I had the toilet brush, my brother the bleach, and mum, the strain. The dry stone wall at the end was too high for me to look over. Mum struggled, hoisting the bucket up to the top of the wall. In the short time that I had known her, I had never seen her pull a face like that. She grimaced and tipped the bucket over the wall.

My brother gypped, my mother gypped and I gypped. Mum took the bleach and poured it into the bucket, swished it around and poured it back over the wall. No one looked over to see where it had gone. My brother muttered something about the bubonic plague, he had been learning about at school. Surely we wouldn't have to do this every week? *"Is this why the country side smells mum"?* piped up my brother. We'd only just scrubbed ourselves clean when the sound of a wagon was heard struggling up the mud track towards the row of cottages. Mum went outside to greet the two men in the wagon. To her horror, this was the Shit Wagon, the very wagon that came every Friday to empty all the buckets and guess what? Our bucket was already empty, and we'd been living there a week. After inspecting our spotlessly clean bucket, mum was grilled on the subject of constipation. They were aware of how long we had been there and were rather amused that 3 people had failed to produce anything between them. Mum's face was blank as the men enquired about how long we intended being on hunger strike as they had a job to do and required results. As they climbed back into their van and proceeded to turn the wagon around, the one with the silver tongue quipped *"when you remember Mrs ...just what might have happened to a week's worth of spoils can you kindly let the professionals know so next week, once your family's constipation is cured, leave it to us to dispose of "*. Mum's face was a picture as the van gently crawled down the lane. The following week the men weren't disappointed as we were made to go as often as possible. *"I want that bucket overflowing for Friday"* she bellowed as I reluctantly skipped across the wet flags to the toilet.

It was cruel to keep kids here, even crueller to keep the rabbit that visited us everyday outside, so mum reluctantly agreed to bring the rabbit in the house as the nights became colder. We got a cage which just fitted under the sink and so all of the rabbit's prayer's were answered as it was allowed to share our dump.

Staring from the front window across the green hills, my thoughts were of dad and our real home. The wonderful scenery fed my imagination as I dreamt up stories of happier times. My young eyes could see for miles down into the village and far away over the rolling fields and down to the town of Halifax in the distance. The chimney tops and mills that dominated the town, stood like pins in the distance. The grass at the back of the cottage was an abundant green that welcomed children to bounce in its softness. It was inches from the cottage due to the slope of the hill. You could touch it from the bedroom window, it was that close. We played in it until it was time to go indoors. We'd ask for our tea outside as it was a lot warmer there but mum would have none of it. The cottage was so run down; it was pointless dusting anything. Mum did her best with a duster, but it was a lump hammer she needed. A knock at the door and we'd be greeted by a shire horse wanting a bed for the night. He'd heard on the grapevine about the rabbit living here and thought he'd check it out. One evening mum tossed a coin to see if we should all move into the outside toilet for a change of scenery and to live it up for a while. As kids we never stayed miserable for long and always made do.

The cottage was overrun with mice. My brother had a plastic baseball bat and his time in the cottage was spent hunting them down. We kneeled on the bed shouting out instructions when we saw one. The rabbit even got into it. He would stand on his back legs, his paws through the wire mesh shouting out instructions. It was a baptism of fire for the poor cat as it was outnumbered and over worked. The cat couldn't keep up with the breeding power of the mice and eventually handed its notice in. Our real home with dad had all the mod cons, wall to wall carpet and central heating, and not a mouse in sight. The house was warm every morning. It was so very different to this place. It was here that I had my first introduction to a coal fire. First thing in the morning, mum struggled to light the damp paper in the hearth. It became the norm to only have a fire in the evening as it was too much trouble. Every morning we froze as we washed our hands and faces in cold water. The water trickled from an old rusting tap that hung over a square white porcelain sink. The cool evenings were spent sitting around the fire. Poking, prodding and feeding it anything and everything, just to keep it lit. On occasion when a cease fire was called, 213 field mice would come out from behind the furniture and gaps in the skirting board and join us by the fire. One of them would play the mouth- organ and another sing and pass around cigars showing us photos of their wives' and children. When the coal bucket was empty mum encouraged us to chip in and fill it up from outside in the biting cold. It must have been hard for mum, taking all three of us away from dad and our warm home but she was trying her best to make this hovel a home. We had some good days and some cold days. Time passed and damp set as ice on the inside of the windows. This was a cold September. By now the mice were enjoying the chase and enjoyed my brother's attention I'm sure they would sit at the windows watching for us coming up the lane. *" Here they come, positions everyone, Brendan, get ready and lie on the trap and play dead, then they won't get the bat out".* The rabbit felt like royalty being taken inside away from cold. I'm sure I heard the mice winding him up saying *"here comes one for the pan!".* The rabbit was the warmest thing in the house. We would fight to cuddle it and I could never get my head around the fact that the rabbit was allowed to happily shit all over its cage in the house and we had to brave the outside toilet. Mum and dad were obviously not getting on and so it was a trial separation. It must have been desperation on mum's part to bring us here.

My happiest day there was in early December. It was now freezing and I came in from the warmth of the cold Yorkshire hills to greet mum who was taking down the Christmas tree. I was baffled and curious, had I dreamt all this? Had Father Christmas been and gone? Couldn't

Santa be arsed visiting this dump? My mind was working overtime; the rabbit was sweeping the pines up while the mice were weight lifting with a bauble before rapping them up neatly in tissue paper and putting them in a cardboard box. What was going on? We only put it up a week ago. Kneeling down in a pile of mouse droppings, mum cupped my cheeks in her soft hands and looked lovingly into my eyes, "We*'re going home, back to live with dad"*. I dived onto the tree and proceeded to pack it into its box at an alarming pace. I was the happiest boy in the world. I hadn't missed Santa after all and we were going home. The mice started to wind the rabbit up. *"Your knackered, they've got central heating down there, you'll sweat your bollocks off"*. I've never seen a rabbit as frightened. He slung the brush into the corner and sulked in his hutch.

A few days later and we were off back to our old house at West Scausby Park, and back to dad. We spent Christmas there and I'd hoped that things were back to normal, suddenly getting up for a pee in the middle of the night was a luxury. I would put my nose up to the window in the night and catch the rabbit rubbing his paws together for warmth, struggling to light his cigarette. I wondered if the mice missed me. Sadly mum and dad's reunion was not a happy one and the sound of them arguing again became a regular thing; even the rabbit had started wearing ear plugs. I'd sit with him in my arms and tell him how unhappy they seemed. I was convinced he could understand and he'd talk back to me. Three weeks later in the middle of January and there was a deep snow fall, the truck came back again, strangely while dad was at work again and we were off once more. *" I'm going to need a new suitcase at this rate" shouted the rabbit "let the mice know were off again"*?

The house was left empty apart from the echo of a broken home, for a second time in a matter of months. I played for the last time in my room as mum ran around in a panic, taking what she needed to set up home elsewhere. It was the end of the road for my family as I knew it. I was only six, but I could feel that life would never be the same again. My worry didn't last as I soon got stuck into what the future had in store.

Chapter 9

STURTON GROVE

Mum and dad's marriage was as good as over. The wagon set off in the snow and I'd hoped it was not back to Bradshaw Rowe .Thankfully we set off in the opposite direction, we arrived at a place called Sturton Grove. The deep snow added to the mystery, I waded up the white path toward the door with the number 23 on. I was hoping that it would be better than the previous shit hole we'd left the mice in. I ran through the empty house, my footsteps giving the house life. I ran into every room with eyes blazing in wonder. The middle bedroom was to be mine. I opened an old cupboard that was built into the wall and found a foot high plastic figure of an ice hockey player, proudly holding his stick. This was a good start; I was amazed how anyone could leave him behind, the house was cold and every room was explored.....I eventually found what I had been looking for. *"YES"* I cried............ an inside toilet!

Mum needed somewhere less damp to bring up her two growing kids. This was the place. I was happy again.

She did her best to furnish the house with what she had, but this place was so much bigger than the one we moved into before. The bits of carpet we had didn't reach the edge of the room. In front of the coal fire it was bliss when it was lit, but behind the settee and away from the warm fire, it was like being in another world. The cold hard floor at the edge of the carpet was an ideal race track for my toy cars. If I was brave enough I would venture behind the settee wrapped up in 25 jumpers, snow boots and a balaclava I was a young Dickie Bird and Chris Bonnington rolled into one. I raced my cars between the gaps in the multi coloured pieces of carpet. The ice cold concrete floor was a perfect track; the black ice complimented my frost bitten fingers. It was a wrench leaving the fire but when a child wants to play, they have to play; and the family of penguins behind the settee took a liking to me and welcomed me into their world.

Between races I would join mum on the settee .We would watch Hughie Green's" Opportunity Knocks" and I'd study the plummets of smoke she gently blew into the room. She would lift her head and stare to the ceiling and delicately empty the contents of her lungs. The blue waves of smoke danced in the cold air and weaved across the room. I would stare at the smoothness of the twisting blue vapours, winding like a snake until it withered away. I was oblivious to the end product. I had no idea that it was the smoke that stung my eyes and tickled my throat, but neither did mum. It seemed that every grown up I came into contact with smoked.

There was no central heating in the house and the only time it was warm was when you were either stood in front of the fire or in bed. When there was no coal left, we would burn anything that we could do without. It

I've Only Got One...

was tempting to throw the furniture on as it had all seen better days, but it was all we had.

On school nights I would fight to keep my eyes open against the heat of the raging coal fire. Eventually the sleep would take over off and I would be sent off up to bed what felt like Alaska. It didn't matter how tired I was, as soon as my feet hit the cold floor, and the frosty air hit my lungs in the kitchen, it might as well have been 2:00pm. I was then wide awake. It was miraculous. It was like being hit in the face with a wok. Bang and the cold got you. The house had three bedrooms but to a young lad it seemed like a mansion. I would lay in bed frightened to death, this big cold house and only me upstairs. Mum seemed to be miles away. *"Night mum"* I shouted at the top of my voice. Time after time I shouted until I got a response. *"Good night...now settle down."* She might as well have been shouting from Burnley, for the confidence it gave me. Three minutes later, *"Night mum"* I shouted at the top of my voice. No answer. *"Night mum"...mum...Night mum".* I was even beginning to annoy myself. The creaking stairs scared me rigid and I would imagine all sorts. Eventually she came up, clad in her own balaclava with a cig hanging out of the mouth hole. She would be firm and instructed me to sleep and stop all this shouting. I wasn't bothered though, it always worked. She always gave in. I would be tucked in nice and tight and have a smoke filled kiss and then be left to freeze my tits off. Her toe would touch the top step and she'd be greeted with another *"Night mum".* I was tucked in so tight that I struggled for breath under the covers. I was too frightened to come out. I would pluck up courage to peep out of the covers and suck in the cold air, then dart back under away from the creaks of the night. When I was brave enough to look into the night, I would see faces in the dark and patterns in the curtains.

I should have written for Hammer House of Horror with the things that went on in my head. Eventually I would fall asleep and wake up next morning with tremendous relief that I was still alive. Even the realisation that it was only the curtains that scared me didn't stop me from being scared to death the next night.

Chapter 10

A CHILD'S NIGHTMARE

It was wonderful being tucked in tight in bed. The only draw back was waking up stinking soaked to the skin and pressed like a sardine in a pool of pee. Dragging my damp body out of the covers was like coming to the end of an army assault course, as I shuffled backwards, with my pyjamas clinging to me. The realisation that I had wet the bed as I opened my eyes and felt the warmth of the wet sheets would break my heart. Mum was furious; I would stand watching as she tussled with the mess in front of her. She wrestled with the drenched bedding. Pulling with all her might until it snapped back and cracked her full in the face. A wry smile from mum greeted me, even though she was annoyed. " Don't just stand there, take your pyjamas off and go and get washed". How come she was so cross, I'm the one covered in piss?

Was there no justice in this world?

My brother never seemed to pee the bed. I wondered if I was some kind of freak. Wetting the bed was to be my secret, although it didn't happen every night, but when it did I felt I had let mum down, I knew she would be angry. If I could climb out of the wet bed, dispose of the bedding and spin the mattress around without her knowing and slide it back in pretending it never happened, then I would. But she was clever, she always knew. Was my brother the perfect specimen? He never seemed to be in trouble, never wet the bed and I never saw anyone hold him down and fart on him. There was certain benefits to being the youngest child, I was always called cute and seemed to get the best cuddle when there was one on offer. These were, however few and far between. I think mum was reluctant to hold a young Albert Steptoe in her arms and tell him she loved him.

My brother was broad and taller than me and usually had a sullen look on his face. He thought before he spoke, where as I never did. I was like a broken record. He would look at me like a father might. He seemed caring but, wary of getting too close to a kid that talked to rabbits and anything that had a pulse. If I ever tried to make him laugh he would fight it but I would know that he was about to crack. But he hung onto the laughter and rarely let it go. It seemed to me that he thought it was a weakness to show emotion of any kind, especially to me. He looked out for me though and with no dad around anymore took on the role of a father figure. He took on a carer's role. He obviously thought he needed to look out for this one. He was a good older brother. He took responsibility for me, he never paid me any compliments, never said anything nice. But when he was sat on my head letting rip with his big fat arse I knew he cared. It was his way of showing me who the boss was. A badge would have sufficed, Instead of his trumping at will. He took on the role of guardian looking out for me; he seemed to grow up really quickly as soon as dad was off the scene. I admired him but didn't understand him and thought he was a serious character. I was usually off in my own world day dreaming and talking to imaginary friends and animals. He was broad, I was thin. He was quiet, I was loud. I loved to laugh; he didn't and would tell me to shut it. I was a dreamer, he was a thinker. I would look at him and want to be like him. I was curious to know why he hadn't any blue lines across his chest, my veins were clear and prominent, naked, I resembled an A to Z road atlas, definitely not Charles Atlas. I was painfully thin and wanted to be as solid and as strong as him.

Once from another room I overheard an aunt discussing my amazing body. *"He's painfully thin you know, have you thought about taking him to the doctors"?* I was ready to burst through the door to defend myself and remind her of my fabulous diet. I was amazed I had a body at all, with the crap I was expected to eat. What was I expected to look like; could she put weight on with a diet of egg bread, toast and jam? By now I was on 12 cups of coffee a day and 20 passive cigarette's. You could double that if I was visiting gran.

I was an expert on all the brands of cigarettes and strong coffee and thought decaffeinated was a kind of injury. Mum changed her brand, depending on price, and as I was now 7 years old I must have looked the part. I was regularly sent to get her cigs. Always served, never questioned by the woman serving on. She must have had a stream of 7 year olds coming in on a Sunday asking confidently for *"Twenty Lambert and Butler and a News of the World please love"*. I even thought about growing a moustache as I felt I finally belonged and I was growing up. As each brand got cheaper, so my order changed. *"Tell your mum we might be doing separate's soon."* The shopkeeper informed me. I got home and passed on the message. *"The woman in the shop said she's separating."* The next 20 minutes were spent describing what she looked like. I looked at her with disbelief as she replied *"she's been on her own for years"*. These adults knew how to confuse. What had all this to do with cigarettes? My rock star diet fed my natural size zero frame, but I hated being thin, my knees were knobbly and looked like knots in string. My eyes were big round and brown, like two polished conkers. There was more meat on one of the chops mum bought from the market once a week. My face was long and with my big chin I resembled a young Jimmy Hill. I was pale and often mistaken for a girl, with my long fine shoulder length seventy's brown hair. I was dressed in anything that mum could afford. Usually it was what my brother had worn two years earlier. Flares and long hair were all the rage and I thought I was a young anaemic Mark Bolan. My elasticated grey flares draped over my 13 inch platform shoes. When I had these on I was a six foot 5 inch 7 year old. Thank the Lord I could see the funny side of things. I knew I looked strange, but what could I do about it. Most kids in our area looked the same. One lad was 35ft tall in his sister's high heels and a midget in his dad's slippers.

Laughter was my friend and I was learning to enjoy it's art. There was something magical in hearing someone let themselves go in a fit of giggles.

I would imitate adverts on the TV to impress mum and her laughter would encourage me to carry on. I felt an enormous sense of acceptance when someone laughed and if I couldn't think of anything funny to keep the laughs coming, I would repeat the line, time after time. A vision of my old pal Cock would appear in my mind and the invaluable lesson he taught me. Laughter had become my distraction and was the remedy for my insecurities.

With the delightful clothes that hung off my coat hanger frame, pale complexion and high forehead, I looked a picture of 1970's nostalgia.

Chapter 11

LAUGHTER

I was now becoming a master at listening in on the big people's conversations. I waited for their chat to turn around to me as it usually did. This time it was Mum and Gran, sharing their cigarettes, both with a full set of teeth in and battling between each other to let the other have one of their fags first. *"Have one of mine…. no have one of mine……no I insist….you have one of mine….no you have one of mine",* eventually one of them took a fag off the other and the story began. It was like a game, a kind of offering, a sort of love gesture. They both seemed to have a box of fags, both with the same amount in each so why don't they just stick their own in their gob and get on with talking about my favourite subject….ME.

I sat in the kitchen and listened as I heard mum telling Gran about the time I came in for tea one evening at our old house. *" What have you been up today then little man"? "I've found a rabbit in a field"* I replied. She explained that my short answer had surprised even her as it seemed to be quite a normal answer. She was for once pleasantly surprised. She prompted me further. *"Did you give it a carrot"*? Trying to humour me, *"No, he'd already eaten, he was 6ft tall, with a big blue hat on and he'd already had his lunch"*. I went on and on, *"He had yellow wellington boots and a suit of armour with the backside cut out so he could ride his motor bike without interruption"*. He'd been fishing with Harold the badger his friend". " Dare I ask what Harold was wearing? queried mum.......holding her breath. *"He was naked........ he's a pervert"* . Mum and gran then took a huge puff of their cigarettes and laughed out loud.

It was good to hear them laughing through the door and cemented my decision to keep laughing at what ever I could. I could laugh at myself and wasn't bothered whether people laughed at what I said or what I looked like. If what I was doing or saying took away my uncertainty or fear, then I was happy to carry on and if I didn't understand something I would laugh at that too. I didn't want to be serious like my brother and I didn't want to be boring like the big people, I wanted to be happy and to laugh.

Chapter 12

NEW KIDS

I missed my pals at our old home and felt a bit alone at this new big house. I often thought about Cock!!! And what he was up to and who he was flashing at these days. Slowly as the heavy snowfall melted, kids started to play out on the green outside the house. We had a porch between our house and next door and I hung around there, hoping to grab the attention of these new kids. Eventually I was approached by a group of them. It was a mixture of boys and girls. Bradshaw and my old home where dad still lived seemed like a life time away, and the kids here seemed so very different. The kids on this street had a different way of talking to the ones I had left behind. They would congregate on the green under the lamppost outside our house or on the park that you could get to through a garden at the edge of the green. Most things happened on the park and I was as green as the grass that covered it. I had heard of bad language but if I ever used any I would be guaranteed a crack. I was lucky to get away with saying pervert, even though I didn't know what a pervert was. There were gangs of kids with an age range of 6 to 16 all knocking about together. Some of the older ones looked as old as dad. They had whiskers on their chins and used words in their sentences that I knew were bad. I had heard some of these before when mum and dad shouted at each other before the doors slammed. Some of these kids were giants to me. Some looked older than dad, but something in the way they acted told me they were not quite grown up yet. I was invited along as the new kid and in their own words *"allowed to "knock about with them "Let's see what you're made of Rat Face"* shouted one of the rougher looking big kids. Today they were playing knock a door run and running over cars.

The whole group set off and I along with the youngest kids was left trailing at the back. The bigger kids stopped at the end of a row of houses and waited for the whole group. Beautifully shaped privets, hedges and fencing stood in our way. On the count of three we were off, one after the other flying through the bushes, over fences and, clambering over flowers and hedges. I looked at some of the smaller kids who looked how I felt. We all had one thing in common, all of us petrified. The kid at the side of me looked like he was pining for his own mum and I felt the same, I yearned for the safety of my front room. But before we could both hold each other and sob, we were grabbed by the bigger kids and tossed into the bush. I felt for this kid with the sad eyes and runny nose as he hung in the air, trapped on a rose bush by the lining of his snorkel coat, waiting to be caught by the house owner. I had no choice but to get the hell out of that garden as quick as my sparrow legs could take me. Another half a dozen or so gardens lay ahead of me and with arses and bodies flying here there and everywhere; it was every kid for himself. Lights came on and doors were opening, there was no turning back. Most of the gardens had high fences on the front and the only way out was across next doors bushes. It was like a scene from the Grand National, the kids replacing horses. Barking dogs helped fill my new beige Y fronts with that day's dinner. They graced the evening sky as my slacks were ripped and hung off my backside courtesy of a passing bush. I began to cry as I ran and ran, with one hand in the air and the other holding the rim of my brothers Y fronts, that mum declared earlier that day were now mine. I looked over my shoulder to see the lad in the snorkel being dragged out of the bushes by the house owner and cracked about the head and yanked this way and that with the hood of his decapitated coat. Those awful swear words were thrust in his face and the more he cried the faster I ran. Eventually I reached the end garden and flew through the bushes, landing on the pavement and boy did I run, I ran and I ran. A few other kids had been caught and were being dealt with by angry residents. Women without teeth shouted and spat and waved yard brushes from their front gardens. All I wanted was home. I walked through the door and mum greeted me *"what have you been doing?"* My hair was stuck to my forehead in sweat, a face full of scratches and my clothes hanging off in shreds, there was no way I was telling her what I had been up to. I knew if I told her the truth, my day would end with a crack. I threw my shredded skid stained y fronts in the wash basket along with my sheep skin over coat and got stuck into a pile of jam sandwiches and a cup of coffee to calm my nerves. Mum didn't press me for an answer as to what had savaged me that evening and left me alone. As I chewed butty after butty and slurped my coffee, I began to wonder where we had now moved to. The kids here were a million miles away from Cock and my old chums so I decided to lay low for a while and play in my room for the next 12 years until my wounds healed and give my mum some time to repair my underpants.

Chapter 13

Six Weeks School Holidays

The months soon passed and the kids still terrorised the neighbourhood.

That first summer was a baptism of fire for me as I witnessed many things and learned lots of new words, usually ones I knew I would get a crack for if I dared share them with mum.

In the 6 weeks school holidays all the kids in the neighbourhood hung around on the park that was surrounded by houses and flats. The park was all grass and was home to two sets of swings, monkey bars and a bell shaped roundabout. It was alive with characters, every one of them older than me. Having lived in Bradshaw for most of my six years I had not heard that many swear words, but these kids knew everyone of them.

After jumping out of bed and deliberately forgetting to brush my teeth, it would be down for breakfast. I was usually the first up and got stuck into rounds of toast and coffee, breakfast cereal was a luxury and I only ever had it as a child if I slept out at one of the posh kids from school. As soon as the toast had passed my lips and the plate was empty, I was out and on my way to the park. It was usually brimming with characters. We would play all day either at football or on the roundabout or diving off the swings. The only breaks came when I heard mum call or my brother came for me or my hungry belly prompted me to go and fill up with more jam sandwiches. One sunny afternoon I was introduced to a new word, well to be exact two, Shag and Shagging.

I was approached by one of the older kids who had no hair on his face, no spots on his chin, and only used words that began with an F and ended with a K *"Rat face, do you want to watch so and so shagging so and so in the bushes"?* Shagging I thought.....this sounds interesting. *"Yes"* I said, not knowing what a shag was, let alone shagging. I followed him to the edge of the park where the bushes had grown wild and were big enough to get under and could quite easily fit three or four people under. Still not quite sure what it was I was about to watch, I was greeted by about six or seven other kids of all ages. We formed a kind of half circle that surrounded the bush. Then it began. One of the older lad's bare bum began to move up and down. Slowly at first, then quick, quick, quick, slow, slow, slow. I couldn't see what all the fuss was about until I spotted someone underneath. A girl's head popped out from under him and had a strange look on her face. Was she in some kind of pain I wondered? My innocence got the better of me and I bent over and looked into her eyes..."Are you alright?" I asked. She greeted my concern with the two words my new mate had the pleasure of using all the time, the ones that began with F and O. How bizarre I thought, and by now his backside was thrusting in and out at a furious pace. *"What's he doing to her"?* *"Shagging her"* came the reply. I bent over to get a closer look and was concerned for her safety and spoke to her again. *"Are you ok"*"? I ignored her bad manners. *"Is he hurting you"*? She didn't reply....she seemed to be in a world of her own. No one seemed to know why he was shagging her, but by now he was going at it as if he meant business. All of a sudden the bare arsed brute gave out an almighty roar as his back and bum cheeks seemed to tighten. *"She's hurting him now"* shouted the lad that invited me to witness the bare arsed wrestling known as shagging. *"Who's winning now?"* shouted a kid smaller than me as he took another bite of his jam sandwich. *"She always wins and he always cries out at the end"*. And on that note the bare bummed brute let out a groan, got up and turned around. All our eyes were drawn to the size and length of the thing that stuck out in the place where his penis should have been. I had seen enough of this shagging thing and made my way back to the swings with the rest of the audience.

A few hours later I set off home after hearing mother screaming out my name, and that my tea was ready. As I walked in she asked what I'd been doing, *"Watching a lad shag a lass in the bushes on the park"*. Crack and as I went flying across the room and sent to bed on the back of her hand, I suddenly realised why people do it in bushes and out of sight. I was utterly confused. Tears ran down my cheeks as I felt an enormous injustice. I had been watching the shagging, I had seen his bare arse go up and down, I knew what I had seen. I had not made it up and I was on the verge of an almighty sulking session. I realised that I didn't want to grow up at all so I decided there and then that I would never shag, it was just too much trouble. If I get cracked for watching, and this was by invite, then what would happen to the lad who was shagging, if he got caught? Still sulking in my room I heard the front door go and the footsteps of my brother coming into the house. Mum was still angry as she began to question my brother about the filth that came out of my mouth. *"It's true mum, he probably was watching it, there always at it round here".* It suddenly went very quiet and the next minute my brother was being chased up the stairs by mum lashing out with an umbrella. I heard him fly past my room and slam his bedroom door shut. Mum shot up the stairs furious that her boys may have had some dealings with shags, shagging or bum bashing. I could not get the picture out of my mind of what I had seen. I lay on my bed and could see the big lads white bum going up and down and straining like a Jack Russell tugging at a chop. I was mighty confused. If it was only wrestling after all, why had they taken all their clothes off and where was the referee? Why wasn't she shouting "submit", she must have been a right tough nut. Next time I go to the park I will ask who had won and why they hadn't worn leotards like on the TV. At times my life was very confusing. What was that thing, where his willy should have been? It pointed at us like a pan handle, maybe they used it in tag wrestling. What ever it was, it looked dangerous and I was curious how it had fur at one end and a slot for pennies at the other. And how come I get cracked and my brother gets cracked and we'd only told the truth. It was another confusing episode in my life that reassured me that the big people were a strange bunch.

Chapter 14

TALKING CANCER

I'm now aged eight and I'm having a strange conversation with mum as we walk to the shops. We were hand in hand, she's doing the usual proud mum thing, wiping my mouth with her hanky and I'd smell the lipstick and sweet perfume she always wears. I always get the impression that I'm not taken seriously by the big people, the worriers as I liked to call them. It was the early seventies and mum was still on her own doing various cleaning jobs. She did shop work and cared for us on her own and never had the time to stop and think that I had it in me to be serious. Where it came from I do not know but I asked her this question. *" Mum, do you think you might get cancer"?* It was a strange question to come out of a seven year olds mouth. She puts my mind at rest and reiterates that it was indeed a strange question for a boy to ask. She was used to me asking lots of questions on all kinds of subjects, but this by my standards was up there with the best of them. My questioning continued, "Well *will I get it then"?* Again I was informed that she is fine and will always be and that I am the same. I cannot remember any other conversation that day, but it has stuck in my mind ever since why might a boy enquire about cancer. The word was a scary one then and still is today. I had heard it somewhere at an early age and associated it with danger, probably off the radio or the TV. What my poor mum thought as I persisted through my questioning I do not know.

Cancer would one day far in the future touch both our life's in different ways, and as the illness came into my life, I was reminded of that moment and wondered if mum had done the same. It does stick in my mind though how odd she must have thought it was for a child to ask about cancer, although with my imagination, nothing probably surprised her. That very imagination has been used many times to mask my fears and insecurities as I've got older.

Chapter 15

COVERING UP THE CRACKS.

I have never had a problem with laughing at myself, its surprising what you can hide or cover up with humour and having the ability to laugh at yourself and at the situation your in. It definitely helps in difficult times. I have found that if you don't take yourself too serious, people will warm to you. Laughter is a fabulous tonic, into adulthood I've stuck to the same routine and it's worked for me. As a schoolboy I talked myself out of trouble with older lads, school bullies could not be bothered with a boy that would slap himself in the face, throw himself on the floor and talk nonsense. They might well have wanted to give me a smack and often did. But more often than not they would shake their heads instead at the tripe that came out of my mouth and then walk off looking for their next victim. Some seemed embarrassed picking on a clown. It was difficult bullying a boy that had the others around them laughing at his antics and it seemed to play with the bullies mind. I would carry on into my teens and adulthood and take with me my weapon of laughter. On leaving school and trying to find work in the early 1980's, I used the same tool. When I was nervous, shy or unsure I would poke fun at myself and cover my insecurities, people seemed to like a pratt that didn't seem to care. When I grew old enough to drink and start going into town, boozing with my pals, Friday, Saturday and Sunday night's, the humour would be a front along with the false confidence that the beer gave me. We had a work and beer culture along with watching your football team and playing at the weekend for a pub team. I've met most of my friends from these pastimes.

The ploy remained the same as an adult, get your one liner in quick as a flash, especially if everyone is drunk and they will leave you alone. The kind of banter that flies around between the "football lads" is crude to say the least. You had to fit in or get the shit ripped out of you. The football and pub banter is reminiscent of my early childhood memories where I learned to try protect myself with laughter. The same friends that would rip you to bits in a group have surprised me and brought me to tears with their kindness and warmth in trying times. When I became ill they touched me with kind words and actions that show that true friends are all in it together. The help a friend gives when you are struggling is priceless and most of them have probably no idea what they have done for me. In time I would realise just how important it would be to be able to talk to people, friends and strangers, anyone that would allow my frustrations to surface and in most cases a good drink would always help to loosen the tongue and tender the heart.

Chapter 16

MY FIRST ENCOUNTER WITH CANCER

At 26 Years old I was still living at home with my Mother and, by now had a stepfather; he had lived with us since I was 14. We were not the Walton's, more like the "Wombles' of Wimbledon Common". My stepfather walked around twittering like uncle Bulgaria and farting about in his greenhouse, he was an amazing gardener. He was what's known as a grafter, but as hard as he worked, the more he would relax and how he loved to nod off in his comfy chair, with his boiled sweets and daily paper tucked down the side, he would not move for the rest of the night. I didn't dislike my stepfather and at the same time I didn't really like him. In time he would grow on me, a bit like one of his prized cucumbers, there were occasions over the years when I would have lovingly chopped one in half and enjoyed inserting it up his rectum while he slept, I'm sure he felt the same about me.

By now my brother had flown the nest and had his own place. Cancer was about to introduce itself to my family. It affected me, not physically, but mentally, as this was my mother's personal encounter. Mum had been going to the doctors quite regularly and as I kept myself to myself I hadn't really taken much notice of why.

I was too busy polishing my stepfather's bald head with methylated spirit while he slept, to think it could be anything as serious as cancer. When I felt particularly adventurous I would carry his sleeping body up to the wasps nest at the top of the garden. If the wasps' stings didn't stir him I would push grapes up his nose, proceed to whack the back of his head with a large stainless steel pan and then measure the distance of the furthest grape. There was an illegal betting syndicate involved and big money to be won on the correct distance of the furthest grape. One time while he slept, I had 25 Peruvian pygmies betting frantically around his chair, he woke to one of them licking his forehead and singing folk songs of home in his ear. Conversations were rare with him. I wouldn't normally get much sense out of my stepfather as he was usually dabbing TCP on his wasp stings with a puzzled look on his face.

On this particular visit to the doctors, mum had been referred to a specialist and it was obviously serious. As I came in from work that night I could sense that something didn't quite feel right in the house. We may not have been the closest family unit in town, and mum wasn't a great one for showing her feelings, but the atmosphere seemed strangely sombre and I somehow knew that something wasn't quite right.

It was as if a dark cloud hung in the air and had taken over the house. I didn't like it but it was too much to ignore. As I approached the kitchen the first thing I realised was there was no meal cooking, the kitchen was silent. The lounge where we normally ate was quiet and no places were set for dinner. I walked into the front room and my family stood in silence. Mum had got everyone in the room and was waiting for me to come home. She was standing there with the strangest look on her face. A look that unbeknown to me, years later I would be wearing. An eerie feel was in the air and I didn't like it, I didn't feel comfortable, had grandma died? Have united sold Brian Robson! I didn't need this, what ever it was I was just a normal bloke, what's happened? What's going on? Is mum getting back with dad? I didn't know what it was I didn't want and was very uncomfortable. The following words seemed to take an eternity to reach me as they left mum's lips *"...I've got cancer!"*. She tried to smile. *"I've got breast cancer!"* I heard the words but they didn't register. Slow motion took over, it was like an invisible cloud that slowed the words down and stopped them making sense. The look on my stepdad's face will stay with me forever. You would have thought he had it I remember thinking; I would later learn that this was a look and reaction that was normal from a loved one. I would in the future witness it once again and then offer sympathy toward him. The people who love you, feel it the most, it may sound a bit of a cliché but it is so true, he felt helpless, close family and friends would rather it be them. When you are the one, you can deal with it. When its not you, you feel helpless, you don't know what to do. You make cups of tea and swap concerning glances with other caring souls and hope your helping.

At the hospital as my mother was told she had breast cancer, she walked through the ward as if she hadn't a care in the world, and my stepfather however had a nurse on either arm helping him out. He took it hard, he cried, mum didn't. People are so very different and when cancer knocks on your door you never know how you are going to react.

Research shows that it knocks on 1 in 3 family doors. It must have taken quite a shine to my small family as it came knocking again, years later. In time it would want the key to my y fronts.

Chapter 17

A SMALL CHILD AGAIN

I stood there in the front room, staring at mum, not knowing what to say. Mum had a helpless look on her face, she was scared and so was I. It seemed to take me ages to walk the few steps towards her and awkwardly hold her in my arms, something I began to wish I had done more of over the years. Her arms were straight and down by her side, she couldn't bring herself to hold me, her youngest son, she was a good honest woman, but showing her feelings was hard for her. I so wanted her to show me some, to tell me that she was going to be fine. It felt good holding her, even though I towered above her, I was still her son and needed reassurance. She was my mum, the mum I had questioned all those years ago about the very same thing that had the power to get a clumsy grown man to hold his mum again.

I stared at the wall behind her as I held her. I didn't say a word; I didn't know what to say. I don't know how long I held her for, it wasn't important; the main thing was that she knew I was there for her. Words can sometimes get in the way. Thoughts ran through me like the time I questioned her about cancer as a boy and how it's come back to haunt me. I wondered if she was remembering the conversation we had. Selfish thoughts darted through my mind of how will I cope if she dies, she's my mum; she was also by brother's mum, my stepfather's wife and my gran and grandad's daughter! It affects the whole family and then there are friends as well.

I was 27 and didn't want to lose my mum, thoughts you would expect from a child ran through my mind. Funny how special my mum suddenly appeared when I realised she may not be here forever. I don't remember crying throughout any of my mum's illness, its funny how the tears have only just started to surface in the writing of this book. I have found you can bury your feelings but they really need to surface, its therapy when they do, at twenty seven I wasn't ready to cry, writing this I now am.

I looked at my elder brother for support, his face was serious, and it was hard for both of us as we never showed any emotions. He was the same as me, cover up your feelings, with banter, and hide them away. He caught my eye and moved his stare towards the living room carpet. I went to my room and sat on the edge of my bed, no music, no TV I just sat there in silence. I was no longer hungry. About a half hour later my door slowly crept open and looking at me through the gap was mum. She had a loving smile on her face, it was clear she was more concerned for me than for herself. What a woman! She asked me if I was alright. I remember thinking "Jesus" she's asking me how I feel and she's the one who has just been told she has cancer. I tried to reassure her that I was ok and did my best impression of bravery for her. I didn't want mum to see me cry. I asked how she was and she tried her best to tell me that she was great and everything would be just fine. *" It looks like they have found it earlier enough , so I should be ok. Once I've been in hospital I will be ok".* I asked mum if she would lose her hair and we both laughed awkwardly. *"Its enough having one bald head in the house with your stepfather"* was her reply. I would have the same question put to me later in my life about my own cancer. This seems to be the first thought of a lot of people when they know you're having a run in with cancer. Mum assured me her hair would be just fine. I don't think she was really sure at that time or not. As mum sat at the side of me and I stared at the floor, we shared one of those child - like laughs. It felt like one of those when as a kid you don't really want to laugh, because you're still in the middle of the worlds greatest sulks and you don't quite feel like snapping out of it just yet. It was a very loving moment, between mother and son. Neither of us knew what it was we were laughing at, perhaps it was the shock but we weren't bothered so we just sat there and laughed. The laughter helped which was the main thing. My life had changed in an instant, mums too. There I was, one minute at work, coming home ready to eat my tea and not really giving mum a second thought and the next, I'm made to realise just how important life and mums really are.

It was a reminder to me just how your mum never stops being your mum. This woman forgives; this woman fights your corner and above all else, never stops loving you. Her soft clothing and wonderful warm motherly aroma had surfaced again. Memories of my childhood crept up on me. I took comfort as a child in her arms and in her hour of need when she probably needed her own mum, she looked out for me. I was now a man and although I was a good six inch taller than her, I felt protected and safe. She sat with me on my bed, caring for me, worrying for me. When really, she had no right as her own health and wellbeing should have been her first priority. Her role as protector and guardian had never faltered. I was an adult, but in her eyes, still needed looking after, even though she was just as frightened and unsure as I was.

The next few days were a blur; the phone never stopped ringing, people calling round to the house. People seemed to look at me differently. Mum's friends would politely smile as if they knew something I didn't, maybe I was just imagining it, but when you're touched by cancer, your whole life changes.

I think the word cancer scares people; it certainly put the shit up me and still does. Some people automatically think the worst; some people don't want or wish to know, not because they don't care, but because they don't honestly know what to do.

A few days after my mum's diagnosis I was booked in for a driving lesson and my poor driving instructor must have thought I was coming down off crack cocaine. I was an absolute mess, I couldn't concentrate, I couldn't get my clutch biting point, the car might as well have had it's mirrors removed for the amount of times I used them. After 10 minutes of screeching and struggling he took over the controls and bollocked me. We had an understanding... he could drive and I couldn't. He was in control.... I wasn't. He was always really direct and I admired him for his approach as it usually knocked me in to shape. He was more like a father to me. It took me two years to finally pass my test so I had probably spent more time with him than I did with my own dad. He knew I didn't like driving, but that day after I chatted to him about what had gone on at home, he took me up to his golf club. This place was special to him and he let me into his world. *"Come on let's hit some balls and sod the driving"*, he said, so off we went. I had never really played golf, but that day, all of my frustration went into hitting those balls. I felt sorry for the man that repaired the windows in the clubhouse and for the owners of the cars in the car park who I hoped had windscreen insurance cover. I felt sorry for my mum and for me and my family and above all for the hang glider who strayed across my path as I connected perfectly with the 3 iron. I hit some beauties and my instructor looked surprised. Every ball I hit was a release of my pent up anger, my frustration at not being able to help mum, my tears that just would not fall and my fear of what could happen to my lovely mum. As I tied a knot in his best club and proceeded to whack it against the side of a tree, he realised that maybe the last few days hadn't been my best.

When he stopped outside our house I began to open up to him and he was an absolute joy. He sat and listened, nodded, and he listened like the father I missed. I couldn't talk to my step father about it; he had his own demons to deal with. But just to release my feelings really helped, he didn't judge, he didn't comment, he just let me open up and it was a tonic. We sat there for a few hours and I felt better, until, that is, the bill from the golf course arrived along with a three hour driving lesson to pay for. It was a good feeling hitting the golf balls with all my might and I'm genuinely sorry for all the ones I lost that day. How strange though that within a matter of years I would be losing another ball of a different kind. This would be one that I couldn't replace by nipping into the golf shop.

Chapter 18

MUMS TREATMENT

Mum went in for her surgery within a few days of her diagnosis and had the cancerous tissue removed from both her breasts. The treatment to stop the cancer spreading would follow once she was over her surgery. Apart from the initial surgery, it's the treatment for cancer that makes you feel ill, unless of course its advanced cancer. Sessions of radiography were to follow and although mum kept her job and finally went back to work when she was well enough. It would eventually prove too much for her so she retired through ill health. Sometimes it's not the strain on your body; it's the mental strain, the hidden scars. It was these that made mum re-evaluate her life. Decisions that may seem major to some, can have little or no importance when life threatening illnesses come knocking. Mum soon left work all together and even though she missed her colleagues and the customers in the shop, she had made up her mind to stop work all together.

Chapter 19

AN INSPIRATIONAL GROUP

Life slowly got back to normal and she made lots of new friends through her illness and became close to ladies that she met at the hospital who had been diagnosed with the same condition. She slowly picked up her life and began attending a group they had formed to help them get back on track. They get together every week on a Wednesday and this is part of her therapy, a choice she made herself and one that's helped her. Everyone is different and people decide themselves what the best cause of action will be to aid their recovery. I am happy for mum and her friends but it was a concept that I struggled with at the beginning. I would poke fun at her and after a few years of her attending the group, I would tell her that she needs to move on and forget the illness. I now know how ignorant and foolish that sounded, but my logic at the time was to leave it in the past where it belonged.

I have since laughed and joked with mum about her group and it's sessions. Even after my own illness I joked that I would set up a group for men that have had testicular cancer. We could all sit around in a circle and a typical meeting would go like this, on introducing a new member! *"Hi my name is Brendan, and I've only got one ball"*. The group leader would ask Brendan to stand up and show the group where his testicle used to be. Brendan would proceed to tell the others that it was his left one that he lost and it used to sit comfortably next to his right one. The circle would politely applaud as Brendan would proceed to point to the scar where his beloved ball once rested and talk fondly with affection about his missing trinket of love.

Brendan proceeded to explain how he tied a small fishing wait to his scrotum and how it now hangs perfectly symmetrical to his body and how it has really helped with his balance. How it has stopped him missing buses, as before he would head to the shelter, just as the bus came round the bend and no matter how fast he ran, he always headed to the right and straight past the stop in the other direction. The group leader would nod and politely thank Brendan. Ralph, another group member would pipe up, and comment from the circle, *"It's a lovely testicle, if you don't mind me saying so, very rounded, you must be very proud?"* Brendan answered with confidence *"to be honest Ralph, If I hadn't have had to have one off I would have seriously considered having one off anyway, it's really changed my life".* Brass rubbings would be a regular feature of the group, each week we could take a copy of "This Week's Ball" news letter. There was a problem one week as we discovered an impostor. He'd been coming to the group for weeks and it turned out he had never had a problem with his testicles, he just enjoyed looking at the other men's. It turned out he had three balls! After we politely showed him the door and Ralph's new steel toe capped army boots, he was allowed to join the week after, now that he met with the correct criteria.

Then it would be my turn to introduce myself to the group. *" Hello, my name is Kean, I've only got one, but it's a beauty!"*

Mum's group continues to thrive; there is a real feeling of togetherness about it. Over the years they have unfortunately lost some of their members through cancer, but the group goes on and so it should. The eldest lady was 85 years young at the last count. Cancer doesn't mind what age and sex you are when it strikes. I initially thought it was morbid having a group connected to cancer and thought mum should let go and leave it in the past. I couldn't come to terms with the fact that people would meet up and discuss cancer, but I'm informed it's so much more. These ladies give each other support and firm friendships have been formed. It really is nothing to do with my initial thoughts about it being morbid, it's about togetherness, having fun together and human spirit, and I'm now hooked. I've met some of the ladies and they are a wonderful bunch. I've even offered to pose for them if they wanted to paint a still nude, thankfully I was turned down.

Chapter 20

HOPE

Mum has been in remission for 12 years. We know how lucky we are to still have her. Apart from the very beginning, when she was diagnosed with cancer, we never sat down and discussed it. In all the years she was dealing with the treatment, the illness and the mental anguish, she just got on with it. It was a very personnel thing for mum. I would soon find this out for myself.

I had hoped I had seen the back of cancer. On buses and in cafes I would here conversations about people being diagnosed with cancer and it always reminded me of how lucky we had been not to have lost mum. It was always at the back of my mind that we could have lost her. I knew we were lucky as a family and I knew I was lucky to still have mum in my life, but I wanted to put it all at the back of my mind and forget about it. I hoped it would be my one and only introduction to the illness. How wrong I was!

Chapter 21

WAS IT GOODBYE LEFTY?

The next time cancer entered my life, it was aimed at me. This time it was my turn! Cancer would touch mum's life again, but in an unexpected way. For now it was her youngest son's turn to realise what she had gone through.

Mum knew what I had to come mentally and I suppose physically. She would see it from my side, but this time and in her own words would feel "Helpless". Seeing her children go through cancer is something she could not predict, this frightening C word had crept up on her family again. This was worse for her as it was something she could not fight herself. She was still in remission and on the way to a full recovery, but now she had to cope with the mental anguish of seeing her son go through something similar.

Cancer was the furthest thing from my mind as I had locked mums experience well and truly away in the deepest part of my mind. I was looking forward to some winter sunshine with my girlfriend who I now lived with. I had been playing Sunday league football, having a laugh with the lads and behaving like most 31 year olds around town at that time. I was physically fit, still had a big nose and was still hyperactive, probably from all the e numbers from the sweets eaten as a kid, thanks to dad at the sweet factory. I had a good job, a career in travel and a lovely home, a crazy male cat called Audrey Maud Knapton and lots of friends. Most of my friendships had been formed through playing or watching football.

It's a Sunday dinnertime and I've just played football. I've gone home and I'm thinking of the latest excuse to get myself out with the lads for an afternoon session on the booze. The usual aches appear the ones that usually go within a couple of days. Nothing more than a good old soak in the bath would fix. The stiffness in my legs and the knocks that I'd taken would pass within a day or so, but I also noticed that I had pulled my groin, probably stretching for the ball. At the time I had had this dull ache for quite some weeks and I just couldn't shake it off. It did cross my mind that it could be serious, but I chose to ignore it. I proceeded to put the thoughts in the room at the back of my mind and slam the door firmly shut. It was the same room where I kept my thoughts about mum.

Weeks passed and the groin ache was still there. My girlfriend at the time and I were looking forward to our winter holiday which was just around the corner. It was not a painful ache, more an annoying one, dull is the best way I know to describe it. In fact I had no pain what so ever. It was just something that didn't feel right. Packing my things for the holiday I told myself to ignore it and that nothing was going to get in the way of a break with my lovely girlfriend. I convinced myself I was fine and nothing was going to stop me from enjoying my holiday.

I had decided to lock it away and forget about it, at least whilst I was away on holiday. I convinced myself the rest from football would sort my groin out and by the end of the week I would be fine.

On the third day of the holiday I was sat on a sand dune, alone as the girlfriend had gone for a cool drink. It was to be the first time I adjusted myself as the discomfort would not go away. *"Maybe it's these shorts",* I thought *"or maybe it's how I am sat or maybe it's heat".* I began to search for any excuse so I could to stop myself thinking of what it might be. I never really thought it could be cancer. For a young fit man to be bothered with cancer was stupid or so I thought. I sat there and pondered. I made a decision, that when I get home I am going to the doctors to get it looked at. I probably have a strain and I'll get some physio.

I thought it was a bit too close to my old balls and the mere thought of a doctor looking at my manhood filled me with dread. I convinced myself again that I would be fine and by the time I get home it will have settled down. SLAM, back in the room the old thoughts went. Apart from the thoughts and the dull ache we had a great holiday and for a time I had forgotten about my fears of going to the doctors and getting my jewels out. I never went into detail with my girlfriend about my fears and the ache as I didn't want to alarm her. She didn't really need to know or so I thought. In the quiet of an early morning it played on my mind. I got up out of bed while she slept and walked alone to the beach. We had been having a great holiday and no matter what I thought of there was no escaping it. The ache was still aching, the dullness still dull, and the fear of facing it head on still prominent in my mind.

The week's sun had given us both a lift, but returning into a cold wet Manchester airport brought home the reality that I could no longer ignore. I had to go and get this dull ache looked at. I had a mental battle with myself, one minute I was booking a doctors appointment, the next I wasn't. It went on and on. After the holiday sun had cooled on my skin and the visa bill was in need of paying I soon slipped into the normality of everyday life. Work, football with the lads a few beers a good laugh and **"DULL ACHE"** still there, still hanging over me even as I laughed. A few days later soaking in the bath and I began to explore where the ache was. I'd seen things in magazines about checking for lumps in your testicles, but never really had the guts to do it, for fear of what I may find. I thought things like this always happened to other people. I looked down and to my horror saw a large brown freckle across the end of my penis. It resembled a birthmark. I had never seen this before in my life and I began to panic. I was scared and in my ignorance I associated moles with cancer from what I had seen in magazines. The mark made up my mind;

I was definitely going to the doctors now. After a few awkward fumbles and the ache still apparent I noticed the roundness of one of my testicles, strangely different from the other. I didn't know what it was I was looking for, but the one on the left, at the side where the ache was, felt different to the other. It was more rounded and it alarmed me. There and then I decided to swallow my pride and visit the doctor. It was to be the single most important thing I had ever done. I was frightened I was unsure but I was determined to get it looked at.

I still convinced myself it would be nothing and it was that thought that gave me the strength to make and keep the appointment. Not for one second did I really believe that it could be that serious. The next morning I rang and made my appointment. A few days later and I would be there, showing the Doctor my privates and it filled me with dread, and it was something I was not looking forward to doing. The fear of the unknown dragged me to the surgery, with my best boxer shorts on and a right good wash of my town halls I set off, apprehensive and nervous. I sat in the surgery waiting for my name to be called out, when a woman I knew, but not well enough to know her name came through the door, I knew she was a big talker and I dreaded her speaking to me. She spoke to the receptionist and plonked herself down next to me. The waiting room was busy and no one spoke apart from the receptionist shouting names out. Why do people sit next to you when you really need to be on your own? She was in the mood for a chat and I wasn't!! *"What you doing here"?* It felt like the whole room was listening, they probably were, I wanted her to leave me alone and leave me with my thoughts. It was like being in one of those small interview rooms in the police station, you see on the TV. She went on *"so come on, what you here for"*. There was no way I was going to discuss my fears with a virtual stranger with half of Europe listening behind their magazines. I fobbed her off with a story about my dodgy knee and proceeded to sit in silence praying for my name to be shouted. What would she and the twenty odd nosey sods in the waiting room have done, had I said at the top of my voice *"Oh I have done some self diagnosis and it appears that my **LEFT BALL** is a funny shape compared to my **RIGHT BALL**, and I have a big brown mole right across the top of my bell end, there you have it."* I'm also scared to death of being here and its bad enough discussing it with a Doctor as well as having you lot listening behind

your Leather and Lace and Fox and Hound Magazines."
THANK YOU".

Unfortunately I wasn't quite brave enough to have said what I was thinking and remained polite and returned the question on how she was in a very quiet voice. The floodgates opened, all I could see was her lips moving. It was to be another lesson; never ask someone how they feel, if they appear to enjoy feeling unwell.

My brain could not register the words coming at me at such speed. I sat for the next 20 minutes and dreamed of what delights I would be having for my tea, after my clean bill of health from my doctor. I would occasionally nod and politely smile, raise an eyebrow, smirk, stick my finger in her eye, pull at her ear lobe and yank at the long thick wire like hair that stuck out from her bushy eyebrows. She went on and on. Her cracked lips told the story of how long she had been ill, how she was off sick, how the doctor had to sign her off and how it's all stressed her out. She'd put weight on and then tried to diet then ballooned again, then tried to cut down on the fags and she ate some salmon which had given her a nasty rash. She'd had tests and she could be diabetic and allergic to fish, etc, etc, etc. I so wanted to take the pan handle out of the old lady's shopping bag and plant the brand spanking shiny wok against her head just to bring her back to reality and to remind her to take a breath between sentences. I was tempted to get my ball out and rest it in her hand as she engrossed herself in her woes. Secretly I wanted to tell her how frightened I was, never the less I remained as polite as ever, just how mum had taught me and smiled. Thankfully my name was finally called out and I made my way to the doctor's room, a quick glance over my shoulder, showed me that she was still talking out loud and had no idea that I had got up and left her. She has now been there 9 years, 32 weeks and 21 days, still without taking a breath.

The moment of truth was upon me and here I was sitting in front of the doctor, about to tell him of my fears, he checked my name and pulled out my file and stared at me from over his glasses. I was at least relieved that it wasn't a woman doctor that I was seeing. Now at 32 years and about 8 months I had only been to the doctors about 3 times in my entire life .Each one with a condition more embarrassing than the last. Here I was again I thought, this time it's my ball, how am I going to tell him about this? I had an idea that the file contained all my past ailments and how embarrassed I felt as he gazed over the notes, pulling some unusual faces as he read about………………

Chapter 22

GETTING A HERNIA FROM THE SUPERMARKET – DOCTOR'S NOTES No 1

I was self-conscious and I had convinced myself that he was reading about the time I was a 16 year old and had just started working in a supermarket.

There were no real jobs in the early 80's just government schemes and I was plonked on to one. I was on a Y.O.P youth opportunities programme. I was a wide eyed 16 year old on £25 a week. I gave my mum £8 a week and £2 towards my catalogue club, where I bought most of my clothes. I always got the clothes over 38 weeks to stagger the payments. By the time I'd paid for one item it was ruined and then the cycle would continue, I'd buy something else and on it went. It was life on the edge. I had a little blue book with all my payments in. On my first day at the supermarket I was issued with a big blue overall that drowned me, but I loved it, I felt like a man.

The overall touched the tips of my catalogue shoes and to complete my look I wore an old mans tie. I walked to and from work with pride, knowing that people could see my overall and think I was a real man, as it hung under my catalogue coat, pure class. At the end of the scheme I was called to the manager's office to be told I will not be kept on, I was heart broken, on the scrapheap at 16. I was praised for 10 long minutes by the two managers before they broke my heart and told me they didn't need me. I didn't cry, but I was close. I thought my career was over and I would never again be allowed to scrape hard chewing gum up off the floor with a paint scraper, whilst the shoppers ran over my young fingers with their dodgy trolleys. I had worked really hard but it was to no avail as another 8 youngsters were released and replaced by another batch eager to impress. It was a sign of the times, there was a ray of hope though. If we ever have any fulltime positions we would love to offer you a job with us, we will definitely consider you. Thank you and goodnight! I took the whole lot in and the two men did seem genuinely concerned for my career or so I thought, it didn't help me though. I was another statistic. All my friends on the same scheme were being told the same, as their 6 months were up they were thanked and moved on, it was happening everywhere. I knew I was special, well more special than the other 7 on the scheme, as I was fortunate to be given a Hernia for my troubles and this became my first note on the doctor's file.

One day I was in the warehouse picking up a box of soap powder and guess who didn't bend his knees? "POP" I felt a kind of tearing sensation in the top of my groin. It turned out I had ruptured myself and although it wasn't evident straight away I certainly noticed in the shower a few days later. As I was showering my magnificent 8 stone frame, like a scene from "Tenko", yes the woman's Japanese prisoner of war camp, I looked down and one of my balls appeared to be missing. Ask any 16 year old day dreamer and he will tell you that it's a bit of a shock when one minute you're masturbating as though there's no tomorrow and the next you seem to have one part of your jigsaw missing. Well I looked everywhere, under the sponge, in the flannel, on the floor, on the shower mat and still I couldn't spot it. Was it in the pink woollen poodle that mum's friend had knitted that held our spare loo roll? Had I lost it on the way home from work? *"Brilliant"* I thought, that's all I need; one of my balls has fallen off. I know I wasn't very sure of myself regarding girls, my body, my fairly new pubic hairs or my spotty acne ridden back, but this was a new one to me. When I get out of this shower I will ring my best mate and see if it has ever happened to him.

It wasn't long before I had found it and I still hadn't got out of the shower, panic over, or so I thought as I realised it had only gone and popped up into my stomach. I felt around the bottom of my stomach and gently pushed the little blighter back down into its sack. While my ball left its sack and entered my stomach, the pain was horrific as if I'd been kicked in the nuts. Every time I forced it back down the pain would go, it was like a game! A game I had no interest in playing. Within a minute of going into my bedroom the little blighter had gone again, followed by the awful pain. I was obviously concerned and informed my mum of my wandering ball.

Within the next hour my mother had proceeded to destroy any street cred I might have had and literally embarrass the pants of her self conscious spotty teenaged son.

She ran out of the house to a nurse who lived in the corner house on our street. The woman and her three kids, all of whom I knew and played with in the street and park marched in to our front room. The next minute I'm lying on the settee with a neighbour prodding my groin, blowing smoke in my face and pushing my ball in and out of its sack, all this with her kids looking on. My underpants were over my knees and I had two woman's heads in my lap and three kids peering over their shoulders. Mum prodded, the woman prodded, the coal man prodded, who let him in? I should have put an advert in the shop window, roll up, roll up, come and push the bollock in and out, up and down, make the spotty teenager scream and win a prize.

After 20 minutes of grabbing and tugging and being told to be quiet, her diagnosis was startling. *" It shouldn't do that"* she washed her hands and off she went, her parting words could have come out of any medical journal *" I'd go the doctors with him, it doesn't look good, it shouldn't do that .They might give him a strap to hold it down"*. My imagination started... a strap , a strap , what the hell is a strap? , I'm 16; I'm not wearing a flaming harness to keep my ball in. My imagination terrorised me. Other people got colds and I get a roaming ball. Wherever I was the little rascal would work himself out of my sack and into the area that caused all the pain, I'd pop him back in, the pain would stop until he set off again on his travels. My older brother was as sympathetic as any 19 year old and would walk in the room with his tongue pushing out his cheek and ask *"Where's it been today then? How high up is he today?"*. Such a caring individual he was then. I had to laugh, if I didn't I would have cried. Mum would tell me that he's only jealous, because his balls never get to go anywhere. I then had a sense of pride that my roaming ball had the travel bug. An operation was to follow and his roaming days were over, they pinned him down and I was pleased that he stayed put. So that was my leaving present from my first job, a hernia and the first note on my doctor's file.

Chapter 23

DOCTORS NOTE NO 2 - IMPETIGO

My next note on his file would read IMPETIGO, this was on my face for goodness sake and all around my eye, it's a beautiful woven outwardly growing crusty highly contagious cold sore type of virus. It has a lovely tendency to seep like honey and where the moisture rests a new one grows. Touch it and touch yourself somewhere else and it starts again, such a lovely condition and yes you guessed it I had it. I was 19 years old by now and my hernia days were well and truly behind me. I was working in a spinning mill. It was a time in my life where it was important to look your best, to attract the girls and to stand out from every other hormone raged teenager. It was all about looking for love.

At that age a spot was bad enough, but Impetigo was in a different league, before it attacked me I thought it was somewhere in Spain. Anything on my face apart from a bit of stubble if I was lucky was a nightmare, a spot was bad enough, and a cold sore was a disaster. The acne on my back was not good, but at least it was covered up, there were so many craters on my back, satellites would circle my head as I slept and NASA would send rockets to test the surface, but Impetigo was unthinkable and so unwelcome. The temperature in the mill where I worked was over 100 degrees and there was oil and fibres in the air. Combine it with a teenager's greasy skin and hormones meant that impetigo was onto a winner....I was the ideal host.

Labouring in high temperatures covered in oil and grease I would wipe my face with greasy hands to get the fibres off as there were no masks provided. It was a modern day workhouse - the place should have been shut down! It was like living in the middle ages, women of 75 were still doing 12 hour shifts when kids as young as me were struggling to find real work. Some of them had been there 30 years or more and if you so much as touched one of their bobbins, they would have you. They had routines and some snotty nosed teenager was the least of their worries I was looked down on as just another inexperienced kid. At 12 noon on the dot an air raid siren would go off right through the mill, on my first day I thought the Russians had come. The siren indicated lunch, this consisted of 30 minutes of freedom and quiet, the quiet was a blessing, like having your ears massaged compared to the previous din of a busy mill. We had 30 minutes to eat and were expected to sit in the filth and fibres that soaked the atmosphere to eat our lunch. There was no canteen so by the time you had taken a bite of your sandwich, it was covered in fibres. Shag Pile Ham was my favourite. The amount of fluff I must have consumed in 4 and ½ half years left me with wall to wall carpet in my lungs and stomach. It felt like I had a small sheep living inside me. I would vacuum my backside rather than wipe it.

The Impetigo loved having me as host, we would go everywhere together , walking in the park, I would strum my guitar to old scabby as he seeped even further down my cheek. I would role my finger across the tender crust and hum a love song, he would then form a circle of crumble around my hand and our love would grow. Working in the mill, I would scratch and rub my face all the more, feeding this little blighter and encouraging him to circle my face. Eventually I could be seen sporting a new crisp balaclava. As the fibres whistled past my highly contagious face it would grow again, this time in another place. It started as a stinging cold spot and grew into a monster. The more I rubbed the more it spread. It would not only cover my delicate skin, but even more annoying it would grow outwardly. After lunch one day, one of the old dears in the mill reminded me I had some biscuit attached to my face. She persisted and was eager to know how come I had made such a mess eating an Abbey Crunch. I felt like a leper!

As another Friday night was upon us the lads were keen to pop to town in search of young ladies. I realised that this was to be one Friday I would not be venturing out, not without my balaclava on at any rate. The lads came to my door to arrange what time we were meeting. I explained that I would be going nowhere as me and the biscuit were staying in and renting a video. They used their usual charm and convinced me that you couldn't tell I had a guest living on my face. They instructed me to cover it in plasters and tell people I had cut myself shaving! I bought into it. I had a bath, read the paper in the bathroom and after vacuuming my rectum I was ready.

An hour later and I looked like an extra from "Carry on Doctor". I was ready for courtship and town. I knew, they knew, we all knew, I looked a tit, they had convinced me that after a few beers and one liners, we would have a ball. Even the biscuit living on my face put a tie on. I was covered in plasters and looked a picture of health getting on the bus; my confidence rocketed as I asked the bus driver to stop staring at the plaster moving around my face. I was willing it to leap on him as we were only feet apart; I was tempted to rub my face against his, just so he knew how it felt. I had spent two hours meticulously sticking the plasters from the corner of my eye over the scab right down to the corner of my mouth, thinking no one would notice. How was I going to find a girl tonight, looking like Chief Sitting Bull.? No one mentioned it, my mates didn't, but I knew what I looked like. I got some strange glances as I walked down the bus aisle to where my mates were sitting. People swayed out of my way, pulling faces and staring at the leper coming towards them. Bits of me fell in the aisle as the bus jerked and knocked me against the hand rails. Wild staring eyes bored into me as bits of me hung off my chin and slowly glided to the floor. I watched the bus driver sweep half of me up in the bus depot and discard me into a bin, I felt the loss, but I would be fine as the impetigo had doubled its mass by now and overgrown most of the plasters lining my face. After a few beers I was fine and almost forgot about my lovely companion, even having a slow dance with him. The odd plaster would fall off into my beer glass, but I carried on, as the alcohol laced my senses I began to feel special and stared into the toilet mirror at my companion. I adjusted my chin and moved a few plasters around and set off back into the night, confident of finding love. At last I had a girl staring at me, she stopped dead in her tracks, had I pulled? The beer was working and I was smitten. She came up close, very close. I felt nervous, my balaclava twitched, she looked drunk, very drunk. She was a brave one or was she just very stupid I thought as the impetigo prepared to pounce. The romantic side of me took over and I began to dream of running away with her, both of us wearing matching balaclavas, spending the rest of our lives together in a mass of crusting sapping soreness. She destroyed my vision, as in a split second she ripped my last and largest plaster off my cheek and unleashed the beast. The pain instantly sobered me up, with eyes popping out and tears welling in my eyes I had had enough. Using my best swear words I told her we were finished, even before we had started she had ruined my plans and It was over.

I sped past her as she was sick on the floor. My mates were all too drunk to notice, I decided to let her keep the plaster and half of my face that was stuck to her cardigan. Enough was enough I was beaten; I walked my living companion home. We stopped for something to eat and I thought about proposing as we were now very much an item. Within a few weeks he had left me and my face, burnt himself out, there was nowhere else for him to cling on to and I was now immune. Oh I do miss him!

Chapter 24

DOCTOR'S NOTE NO 3 - PILES

I had only visited the doctor on one other occasion, this was to be an experience equally as embarrassing, this time It was piles or as written in my doctor's words, "haemorrhoids". I knew something was not quite right as the carpet had taken on a strange redness. I noticed this whilst hoovering up my back passage one day after work. *"Oh dear"* I thought, I had better make an appointment at the surgery. No wonder I dreaded it when I had to make an appointment with the doctor. I had to take off my trousers behind yet another curtain and lay on my front. *"Oh bloody magic!"* I thought as he prodded around. I was diagnosed with bleeding piles and given some pile cream and a barbaric looking contraption. This was to glide the cream battleship missiles up my passage and change the colour of my carpet. I could see him reading my notes as I gave him a gentle smile.

I knew what he was thinking, "Hmm, three visits, **HERNIA – IMPETIGO – PILES".** He sat for a time, slowly running his fingers over his chin. He seemed frightened, fear was etched on his face and I tried to read his mind. *"Oh no not him again, why do I always get this bloke"?* We sat in silence, him looking at my notes pulling strange faces and me looking at him, as If I was somehow proud of my records. Thoughts ran through my head on how it's always my backside, my testicle or a highly contagious rash when I come to the doctor's? I thought about all the doctors getting together in a morning looking at the list of patients names and then mine popping up. I was the short straw. I remained still in my chair, waiting for him to speak. I remained polite, again like mum had taught me, but I felt like a freak. I'm sure he was dying to ask me why I never have a cold or something normal. I began to think he thought I enjoyed pulling my trousers down in his office, that I got some kind of kick out of it. So there it was three visits, each as embarrassing as the last. Now I'm here on my fourth visit, my hardest one yet and I am sat waiting, frightened, nervous and dreading telling him. *"What appears to be the trouble Mr Turner?"* As if he didn't half expect what was coming? I knew what he was thinking, *"I hope it's not his genitals again".* As I began to tell him that I had a mole on the end of my penis and would he mind looking at it, his face was a picture. *"On the end"?* He repeated, really slowly. His fears were confirmed!. I'm sure he reached for the panic button under his desk. He instructed me to take my usual position behind the curtain and take down my trousers. Three out of four visits to see him had ended up with my pants down.

The old familiar smell of rubber gloves was in the air and I was being examined again. I continued about the mark on the tip of my penis and he was not too concerned about it, even though I knew I had never seen it there before. He dismissed the mark as a freckle and that it was absolutely fine and weeks of anguish lifted with his words. *"It's just a freckle, nothing else "* I felt alive again and sorry for wasting his time. Relief ran through me, thinking I was ok to go. He asked me about any discomfort that I might have and assured me to forget about the freckle. I could sense the seriousness in his tone and I began to explain how long I had felt a dull ache. I showed him where. As I stared at the ceiling he examined me, his words then ripped into me. *" I am concerned about your left testicle"* as he carried on examining me. He told me that he was going to refer me to a specialist at the hospital. I had gone to the appointment alone but now wished I had my partner with me for support, I didn't expect to be told I was being referred to hospital. *"What are you sending me to a specialist for"?* I asked, *"You need a full examination, I want to be sure your left testicle is ok"*. He reassured me and told me not to worry and tried to put my mind at rest, but it was too late. All sorts of thoughts were going through my mind. His examination then moved to my back and my neck and he questioned how long I had had the dull ache. His questions fed my imagination and I began to think it could be more than just a groin strain. I wanted reassurance that I was going to be fine. I questioned him that the mark was a freckle and not a cancerous mole and again he put my mind at rest. *"If I'm fine and it's a freckle why do I have to go to the hospital"* I asked. He went on *"I need to be absolutely positive that it is nothing so that's why I need to arrange for you to attend a hospital appointment"*. It was the freckle I found that made my mind up to visit him in the first place and not the dull ache. It gave me a bit of a chill. If I had not found the freckle what might have happened to me? This always sticks in my mind. I would not have had the courage to visit the doctor in the first place, let alone have an examination. I was instructed that I would be sent for by letter. I left his surgery in a strange mood not sure what it was I had just heard and began to worry.

A few weeks later the brown envelope landed on our doormat. It looked official and serious. I was to attend an appointment in a few days time at The Halifax General Hospital. Apart from the dull ache I felt fine and had tried to put my little dilemma out of my mind. I was to visit hospital and have an ultrasound scan; this was to be a strange experience. A middle aged man instructed me to undress and invited me to lie on the bed. He then introduced my testicles to a cold gel. He ran a hand held device all over my privates. The cold slimy gel was not very comforting for a confused state of mind. My eyes wandered around the small room, more through embarrassment. I examined the door frame, the cracked paint in the corner, the plastic light above my head with the dead fly's and the boring looking poster on the wall. His gentle tone tried to reassure me that all he was doing was routine and I was going to be fine. As I began to worry the ice cold gel turned into a tonic to my sweating genitals. Thoughts of why oh why and why would anyone wish to do what this man does for a job. How he must have told his careers officer 40 years ago that he wanted to rub cold gel in men's privates and then get paid for it. He kept trying to break the embarrassing silence until I asked him if he had a preference to left or right testicles. He didn't bat an eyelid and replied that they were all the same to him. We chatted and he explained that he had just about heard all the jokes there could be about his chosen profession. All the time he concentrates on the black and white monitor in front of him, looking for anything abnormal. He smiles and answers my questions and laughs when I enquire about getting the football results on his monitor. *"No, I'm afraid its just spot the ball today"* and we both chuckled. I could tell he was a kind man, just like all the staff I was to meet on my journey. He was clearly comfortable at putting young men at ease in a somewhat awkward situation. He assured me he hadn't found anything. After more intense questioning from me, his answers were now becoming one word so I decided not to ask him anything further. I was left to clean myself up so I then left the room with my boxer shorts clinging to my thigh. He instructed me that I would receive notification of my next appointment, where they would discuss the results of the scan. I walked back to my car with an uncomfortable feeling, sticky and uncertain, not sure of what was happening to me and what he had been searching for on the monitor.

All sorts went through my mind as I left my new gentle friend and squelched to my vehicle, will I smell on the way to work? I felt like a freshly cracked oyster, Will the jelly set? Will my groin become entombed in a crisp shell? , will the man tell his wife about my questions and how small my penis is?

Back at work I joked with a colleague about having the jelly you find in pork pies smeared over my balls and the strange experience I had just encountered. As I talked I thought maybe I'm saying too much, but as we both laughed I found that it helped to discuss it, and it helped even more to see the funny side wherever I could. The fact that I had been followed to my car by a pack of starving stray dogs sniffing at my groin hadn't bothered me in the slightest. Other people at work in passing asked where I had been all morning. I think my answer surprised them and as I was still in a light hearted mood about my experience *"I went to meet a middle aged man who rubbed jelly on my privates"*, they laughed *"you never get any sense out of him."* I was being honest, I did feel awkward, it was all new to me and I didn't wish to tell lies but I also didn't know how best to deal or how to discuss it, other than with brutal honesty. Some colleagues thought I had a vivid imagination. Rumours had however spread that I was now seeing an escort worker who lived and worked on a jellied eel farm.

Chapter 25

FINDING OUT I HAD CANCER

Two weeks later I received another appointment letter instructing me to attend an outpatient's clinic at the same hospital. This was for the results of my scan. The day of the appointment soon came; it was a grey bitter November morning. My partner came with me for support; she seemed more concerned than me. I thought I would be in and out and back to work in no time. I had no idea of the life altering diagnosis that waited for me. Although I was surprised at the speed in which I was being referred from one appointment to another. I was nevertheless unprepared for what lay ahead.

The waiting room at the hospital was as dull as my ache. Row upon row of old school house plastic chairs waiting for patients and loved ones bottoms to grace. An 11:30 appointment was seen at 12.30pm and the sign on the wall that greeted you on your way in gave you some idea of the wait ahead. *"We are running precisely 1 hour behind schedule today and your patience is very much appreciated"* The complaints were coming thick and fast from the waiting masses. The staff remained calm under pressure as people demanded to be seen. It was clear that the nurses knew how to deal with the complaints and had probably seen and heard them a thousand times before. Still blasé, I sat there, my mind empty, staring around the room. Boredom was my companion as my partner sat reading the paper back to front. I had convinced myself that after this appointment I would be done with hospitals and get back to getting on with my life. It resembled a cattle market and the cows wanted out and home to their fields.

"Do you know how long I've been waiting "? cried out one middle aged man. Others looked at their watches as if their lives depended on it. God forbid if someone got their name shouted out before you if they had not been waiting as long. I tried not to be bothered and did my best to remain patient but it was getting to me. I had a numb bum from the plastic chair and was getting fed up of hearing people whinge, the coughing and spluttering was starting to affect my patience. The atmosphere felt tense. Strangely, listening to these people helped to pass the time. We passed the morning paper to the man across who seemed as keen to get out of there as I was. Finally I got the call, my name was shouted out. Now I was ready to get the hell out of there.

My partner stayed in her chair as I reassured her that I wouldn't be long. I left her looking worried. I didn't think I would be that long, after all I was just getting some results and then I would be away. Whilst I had been waiting I had noticed that other couples had gone into their appointments together, never the less I still went in alone. I thought I was a man and I could deal with this, whatever it was and deal with it alone. I soon realised I had made a mistake and had made the wrong decision.

I was taken to a cold whitewashed clinical looking room. I could see a patch of green grass through the window in the distance. I wanted to be sat on that patch of grass and away from here.

Two chairs fed a table and a door to the side led to another room. There was no bed, at least I didn't have to lie down and take off my trousers yet again. This was a good sign. I waited as instructed by the nurse who assured me the doctor would see me in a few minutes to discuss my results. Fine by me I thought, in and out and then off we would go as it's the weekend tomorrow. I have things to do.

Another 15 minutes and the doctor finally came in through the side door; he introduced himself and didn't seem much older than me. He read my notes looked deep in thought and then made some comment about the waiting time and vanished again through the side door. By now I was getting a little concerned, I was thinking that if it was really nothing, then why am I still here. I had picked up on the fact that this doctor who vanished was liaising with someone else in the other room. I thought about my gentle gelling friend and his assurance that I would be fine and started to doubt that he knew what he was on about and that maybe he could be wrong or maybe it was his job to reassure people, after all he had a kind face. The side door opened again and it broke my thoughts, it was the doctor again. He leaned against the table and asked if I had come to the appointment alone. I told him about my partner in the waiting room. His next sentence cut through me *"I think it would be good advice to ask her to come in and join us as we discuss your results"*. Masses of thoughts flashed through my mind, I think I was then in a state of shock, this must be serious, what did it have to do with my girlfriend?

This was the first time I felt out of my depth, I was frightened and confused. It didn't feel right; my eyes darted around the room I was trying to make sense of what he was saying. I couldn't focus on anything, as I slowly got out of my seat and set off to get my girl. My humour had betrayed me. As I walked over to her she met me with a beautiful smile and put down the magazine she was now reading. *"Are we going"?* She asked *"no they have asked me to come and get you, I think they want you in the room while they discuss my results"* Her face dropped, she was a nurse herself and had picked up on the fact that something was not quite right. Her eyes met mine, there was no smiling now. The small walk back to the room seemed to take forever, I felt like the whole waiting room was looking at me. We sat in the room waiting for the doctor to come back in. She held my hand tightly, I shrugged my shoulders and raised my eyebrows and tried my best to reassure her, but I didn't have a clue what was going on. I tried to smile but my eyes said it all. She wasn't stupid; we sat there in silence, hands clamped tightly together, both trying to make the other feel better.

The doctor came back in, I'd got the impression something was not quite right. It was as if he had to keep going into the other room to check the notes and prepare himself for the news he was about to break. He started to talk looking at both me and my girl, we looked up at him, as he was now perched on the table edge. *"I'm afraid we have found from the ultrasound scan that we are almost certain that you have a malignant tumour. We will have to remove your testicle and sperm ducts. We will then send it to the laboratory for histology, to see whether or not you need any further treatment. This would consist of either chemotherapy or radiotherapy"*. I'm sure if I had understood the words he had just spoken, I would have fallen flat on my face. The only thing I remember taking in from his sentence was that he was going to remove my testicle, remove my testicle, remove my flaming testicle – what for? I looked at my girl, I looked at him and I looked at the white wall behind him. *"Hang on a minute, sorry if I sound a bit daft here but, you said something about removing my testicle?!"* *"Yes we believe you have testicular cancer"*. CANCER, losing a testicle, it didn't register. Thank goodness my partner was with me in the room, she took most of it in. Here I was thinking I would be back at work in an hour or so, with nothing to worry about and now I'm being told I'm about to lose a testicle and could have cancer. He left us alone for a while and we just sat there. I stared into space, I was agitated and confused. I kept repeating "I've got CANCER, CANCER," and I'm going to lose my ball. *I didn't expect that"*! Tears began rolling down my partner's cheeks; I wiped them away with the palm of my hand and didn't know what to say to her. The 10 minutes we were left alone in the room were the strangest. I didn't know what I was doing or thinking.

Within the hour I was sent for blood tests and chest X-ray's at the other end of the hospital. We walked to the Blood Department, up through the long cold looking corridors. *"What about work"?* I said, *"What about letting them know, how long I've been?, I had said I'd only be a couple of hours"*. My girl reassured me, but by now my mind was racing. Thousands of thoughts battled to be the first to come out as words. *"I'm going to be a eunuch, a eunuch"*. I repeated it all the way up to the Blood Department, eunuch, one ball, Hitler, eunuch..... eunuch....eunuch. It started to sink in. I went on a rant. *"Your boyfriend's a eunuch, this can't be happening. Can't*

I get flu like normal people? I don't get flu me, just take my balls off." My poor girl was getting it in her ear all the way up the corridor. *"Eunuch Turner, that's me",* I had suddenly become obsessed with the word EUNUCH.

As we sat in the waiting room listening out for my name to be called, a man came in with filthy overalls on. He acknowledged us and I couldn't help but smile at his dilemma. The bloke didn't seem particularly bothered about his mishap but it looked quite serious to me. He had a piece of wood stuck to his hand by a drill bit. I couldn't help but smile, he was obviously in shock as he didn't seem at all fazed by the cupboard connected to him.

They called my name out but I insisted they see to the human wardrobe first. He thanked me and off he went. I thought it was more urgent than my case. My partner told me off *"You've just been diagnosed with cancer and you're letting someone take your turn in the queue."* The strain was starting to show and I was still in shock. I snapped back." *He's got half of his workshop hanging out of his hand; I think I can wait a bit longer".* At the time I felt luckier than the walking wardrobe. It hadn't kicked in yet what I had been told. Maybe I didn't want to know what was really wrong with me; maybe I was hiding the truth from myself.

Fifteen minutes later they brought the wardrobe out on a stretcher, it was in bits! The drill came next, a bit screwed up, followed by the bloke, a lot lighter and a lot whiter. I think the shock of what he'd done to himself just hit home. He said his goodbyes and left, just like my ball was about to. My eyes wandered around the white walls. I stared for a second, moved my gaze and stared again. I was sombre, my girl was with me, sitting real close, next to me in fact, but I felt so alone. Was this it, was I going to die? It felt like no one could help me, I stared at the receptionist, I stared at my feet and I stared at the passing porters. I was well and truly in my own world. One minute I felt sorry for myself, and then I didn't, my mind was racing. I felt so very strange and so very lost.

I had planned to be back at work by now with the dull ache in my past. My chin touched my chest as I slid deeper into my chair. I wanted to be alone, but I also wanted to be held. My pride got in the way of asking for help. I was being selfish. She was trying to be strong but must have felt helpless. Thoughts came like rapid thunder, what could she do? What could we do? What could I do? I turned my head to break a smile in her direction and she gave me a half one back and held my hand. A tear stuttered as it gently rolled down her cheek, it weaved down her tender smooth skin and vanished as it caressed her lips. The second tear was quicker than its sister, the whole family then appeared. I knew she was trying to be strong, trying not to cry, but it was no good. As she wept, she whispered *"We're going to be alright aren't we? What am I going to do if I lose you?"* *"I've just said that to my knackers"* was my swift reply. She wasn't in the mood for humour, but it was all I knew... It was so very quiet in the waiting room .I was embarrassed but I held her and spoke *"I'm going nowhere and not to worry"*. I didn't know where the words came from; I was scared but knew I had to reassure both of us, that things were going to be ok.

I tried my best to reassure her, I didn't know who I was trying to reassure her or me. I knew I had to be strong for both of us. It was starting to hit home. By now I had hoped to be at work with the appointment behind me, and not in another part of the hospital having my bloods taken for the first time and then the first of many X-rays.

It was a blur, surreal; things like this don't happen to me, they happen to others. Every now and again I would hear in passing that so and so has cancer; you grimace, feel for them, walk away and then put it to the back of your mind. Now it was happening to me and I would be one of those people, the kind that people talk and look at differently, as I am now a CANCER sufferer. I felt I had been labelled with something that singles you out, sticks you in a group, a minority that people are scared of. I felt part of a group that stops to make you think about how fragile life is. Thoughts that normal people don't want to think about. I used to think the same. I had switched groups. I was now labelled. I started to feel odd. Thoughts flew around my head like shooting stars across a murky sky. Why have I got cancer? Why me? What's wrong with me? Why does it have to be in my testicle for God's sake? Of all the places and how am I going to tell people, I'm a Eunuch, will I still be a man? I don't feel ill, I'm not ill; maybe they've got it wrong. I wanted children one day so now what? Can I have them? What about my partner, this could affect everything. What will she want with a bloke with one knacker, a eunuch who fires blanks? My mind was again working overtime. I felt dirty and different.

It was now more than an hour since I was told and I was starting to realise that this was really serious. I didn't cry, I don't know why I didn't cry, we weren't brought up to cry. I began to wish I could cry. I was called for my chest X-ray and the lady was very kind. *"Shirt off, arms down by your side"*, she popped out of the room in a flash, *"next one, arms in the air, stand still"*, popped out again and flashes. *"That's it, you're all done."*

Next was the trip to Bloods. I'm not a needle man, but I was that numb from my news they could have taken it out of my chin and I wouldn't have complained. *"Don't worry"* said the nurse *"Its very quick",* she was right, it was clinical and all done in minutes. I looked away while she looked for a vein. I pinched my thigh to concentrate on**,** rather than the needle about to go in my arm. I couldn't feel my leg, what's happening to me? The nurse then politely but firmly instructed me to stop nipping her thigh. *"All done, you can go now",* "home?" I replied, " *yes"* said the nurse

Chapter 26

A WAITING GAME

It was now a case of waiting to see how advanced the cancer was. I was starting to think about not wanting to lose a ball, but I didn't want it connected to me, if it's cancerous. We drove home and I rang work, and told them I had just got out of the hospital and that I wouldn't be long. Funny what you do when you've had unsavoury news. I had a cuppa with my girlfriend, gave her a cuddle, and told her it would be ok, wiped a few more tears from her eyes and went back to work. I apologised to the boss for being late back and then tried to get on with my work.

At that time I worked for a travel tour operator. Our department was responsible for contacting guests and travel agents to let them know of changes to their holidays, cancelled flights, overbooked hotels, and building work. The Calls we received were usually negative. People shouted and screamed at you over the phone, they needed someone to blame if their holiday was ruined or altered. I was in the firing line and dealt with calls of this nature. I tried to forget the news I had just received by concentrating on work. I later realised that I was crazy to go back to work straight away. I felt I had to ignore my news and carry on with my life, I was in shock, but I didn't know at the time. I picked up the phone and dialled the number of a travel agent to tell them of the change to their customer's holiday. They had been moved from one resort to another and downgraded from a 4 star hotel to 2 star apartments. I gave the travel agent the news and she started to chew my ear off, cursing this and cursing that. *"You cannot do this; this is one of my priority customers, they book every year and have 3 or 4 holidays a year".* She was concerned for her passengers and rightfully so and was not in the mood to listen to my usual calm advice on what options she had and the reasons behind the change. It was about now, that I realised just what it was, that I had been diagnosed with, only two hours earlier. She was ranting into my headset, *"What are you going to do? How can you do such a thing? How can anyone do your kind of work?"* she was getting personal and I was her target.

I wanted to tell her I had just been diagnosed with testicular cancer. I think I was still in a state of shock. The phone slammed down at the other end and I fell into one of my day dreams. I tried to type notes into the computer screen booking and write down the details on the manual file, but my head was having none of it. I dug really deep to try and stay focussed and positive. I looked at my watch; I had two hours to the end of the day. I willed myself to get through it. I pondered on why I allowed myself to take this crap about a holiday from a travel agent, when I may not be here for my next one.

My supervisor spotted me staring into space and asked if everything was ok. She enquired about my hospital visit. I froze on the spot.

"They told me I have testicular cancer and I've got to have surgery". Her jaw dropped. It was the last thing she expected to hear. *"Oh I'm so sorry".* At that point in time she was the first person other than my partner to hear my news, her reaction frightened me. She sat at the side of me *"Oh no, oh no, not cancer are you going to be alright"?* I didn't speak, I just shrugged. I knew that if I spoke my voice would crack and I was beginning to feel emotional, it had been a long day.

My inner voice cried out ....for God's sake if you're going to cry mate, save it for home, don't do it at work in front of all these people. She was amazed that I had even thought about coming back to work, let alone coming in and just getting on with my job. I told her about the rude travel agent and that it nearly tipped me over the edge and she was genuine in her compassion. It meant a lot, but it also brought it home how serious this could be, just by her genuine concern and reaction. She asked me to go home, but I stayed, and put on a brave face and tried to be as normal as possible even though I was beginning to feel like I was going to crack.

Within a week, I received the first of many brown envelopes that would drop through my door, the customary Doctors hospital appointment. I had to go and see my GP to find out the results of the X-ray and the bloods taken, this was to be the following Friday. This time I made sure my girlfriend came in with me. I was told about the type of tumour, they didn't mess about, I was advised that I was to be admitted the Tuesday of next week and I would be going in for surgery. This time next week I thought *"I will be a Eunuch".* I didn't really know what a eunuch was, but somewhere in my life I had picked up on the fact that Eunuchs' had no balls. It hit home, two balls Friday, one ball Tuesday, oh dear, oh dear, oh dearie me , I tried to laugh with the doctor who had probably heard and seen this kind of thing a thousand times before. He explained the procedure, how many days I will be in hospital and how I might feel. He advised me of the healing process and of how long it might take. He told me I would be having a high dose of chemotherapy once I was fit again, after having the surgery, to remove my testicle. This was to be about 4-6 weeks after my operation and would hopefully clear up the cancer once and for all. Although the tumour was in my testicle and would be removed, the chemotherapy would kill the white cells and take away any cancerous cells.

I was amazed at the speed of my admittance to hospital. There had been hardly any time since the original diagnosis. After receiving my blood results and the knowledge from the markings and the depth of the tumour, I was now in the thick of it. They don't mess about. I wasn't looking forward to parting with my left testicle; but I also wasn't too chuffed about carrying one about that contained a tumour. If they don't move quickly, or you are not diagnosed soon enough the cancer can take hold and work its way inside your body. I realised just how lucky I was. At the time I didn't feel too lucky, but over the years I have gradually got used to the situation and thanked my lucky stars for my early diagnosis. Had I ignored my dull ache, who knows how far it would have spread? Before I never gave a thought to checking my balls, thankfully most of my friends now do………… some of them even check their own!

When cancer touches someone close it makes you realise it can happen to anyone. One of the lads who is quiet and can't stand the Doctors has been in regular contact with his testicles. He tells me they now have a lovely relationship. He regularly roles them between his fingers, he's now sold his worry beads, who needs them when you've got a lovely pair of conkers to take your mind of your worries.

I hear countless stories about people I know that have now taken the time to regularly check themselves. Some have gone to their own GP after finding lumps and thankfully they were only cysts, lumps of fatty tissue. Thankfully within my circle the message to check yourself seemed to be getting through. It takes a brave man to look for something he doesn't want to find and a braver one who has the "balls" to act on it, if there is something there. I'm glad I've talked about it, I'm glad I've laughed about it and I'm glad my friends have listened. It's also helped me to work through some of my demons and pain. I might have looked like I didn't care, but I did and laughter is a great substitute for anger it also disguises many fears.

Chapter 27

LAUGHTER AND HOPE

Laughter was also a beautiful mask to wear at a most difficult time. When I was laughing with friends, it was a kind of therapy. It helped and still does. It releases hope and allows you to enjoy the moment. I've been frightened, and cancer can remind you that we are not here long enough. It reminded me to enjoy what I have, not to look too far into the future, and not to spend too much time dwelling in my past. Enjoy the present moment, enjoy today, and enjoy my family, my friends, not to take life too serious, spend time with my imagination and smile.

On the day of finding out I had cancer, and after I left to go back to work my girlfriend phoned everyone we knew. I was doing my best to put it to the back of my mind but she had other ideas. At the time I thought she had told the whole world I was losing a testicle and I was losing my masculinity. I didn't really want to tell anyone at first as it was still sinking in. I was struggling coming to terms with living the rest of my life with one testicle.

I hadn't planned my next move. I hadn't thought about how my family and friends might feel.

My partner's way of dealing with the news was to tell people. It's easy to forget how it can affect people close to you. It helped her deal with it; I tried not to deal with it so head on and hid most of my fears from people. That day as I returned home from work the phone never stopped ringing. People I hadn't spoken to for ages were concerned asking how I was.

Then mum called, I told her I was fine yes, a little confused and that I didn't feel ill. My mum wanted to help, she'd been there before, seen it, done it, now it's her son's turn, she was very supportive, and told me that if I ever need to talk she'd be there for me. I never took her up on that, not that I wasn't grateful, but I would try and sort my own head out and she probably knew I needed time. She felt helpless. Cancer was again in her life, but this wasn't a battle she could face head one, like the one she'd got used to dealing with. Cancer had now appeared twice in her family, once to her, and now to her youngest son.

Chapter 28

WE'RE ONLY HUMAN

At the beginning I took the diagnosis personally, something I had to deal with alone. I used to think it was my problem and mine alone, but it's not. People that care about you can feel helpless and can suffer just as much, but in other ways.

By the end of the night I was sick of telling people I was fine. I put the phone down after another call of support and lost it. I raged at her *"what have you phoned everyone for? Why not put it in the local paper. I'm losing one of my knackers".* She'd done nothing wrong, but it felt like she had gone through the phone book and told everyone about me, not being a man anymore. It had been a long strange day, for both of us. I was very annoyed, *"I'm sorry"* as she said it, the phone started ringing again." *Who's that, Terry flaming Waite? You better answer it as it might be NASA wanting to fly around my bollock!".*

It had been our longest day yet. I didn't need this, another call, another bloody call, people I hadn't spoken to for years. *"I'm so sorry, how are you? Are you going to be alright?"* I felt I was in the headlines, I know my partner meant well but it seemed the whole world new about my business. I cracked open a tin of lager and off it went again, ring, ring, it was my dad, this time, *"oh son",* he sounded concerned. She had started an avalanche, she'd phoned her mum, my mum, her sister, my brother, they had then phoned someone else and so on, - the Vatican was engaged fortunately for me and for the phone bill!

I knew I was having my surgery on the following Tuesday so I had the weekend to think about my situation. Friends popped around to see me and they genuinely felt terrible. The crazy thing was that I felt absolutely fine. I didn't really know how I felt, as I felt well within myself, just scared and uncertain. I went for a pint with one of the lads the day after and it hit home just how awkward I felt.

People seemed to be looking at me differently. In the pub someone patted me on the back, gave me a cuddle, and said sorry. Some appeared to be looking at me as though I had two heads. I escaped to the toilet and smiled to myself in the mirror above the urinal. As I began to pee for England I spoke to my doomed testicle...I cupped him in the palm of my hand, just like grandma did with her budgie, *"Do you know left knac what trouble you have caused me?"* He looked up and twitched his acknowledgement, it was a moving moment for both of us, and it was to be one of the last times I held him.

I put my bravest face on and pushed open the toilet door with my now locally famous crutch. I told myself to keep smiling, and enjoy a few beers with the lads. If I have a laugh, I can get through this. Word had gotten around amongst the boozers about rat face and his soon departing bollock. I wasn't prepared for the drunk in the corner though, *"why don't you have them both off and I can take you out darling"* You'd make a great bird, with your skinny little legs, it's a shame you've got no arse though". I never did take him up, he wasn't my type, but his beautiful words lit up the room and made me feel so special. *"When you've had your bollock off, I will come and see to your lass"* then she can have a right pair of balls slapping against her thighs instead of just the one". This was supposed to be a friend of mine. Then up he got, bought me a drink and cuddled the living daylights out of me.

Chapter 29

GOING FOR THE OPERATION

Tuesday came quickly and I was on my way to hospital with my bag in hand. Packed neatly.... It's amazing how you suddenly acquire a pair of paisley pyjamas and a dressing gown, all my adult life I had slept naked. My Manchester United slippers had even been scrubbed with suede cleaner, my partner had thought of everything.

I was admitted to a small ward with four beds that would in time be shared by three other men, all with different conditions. The room was as clinical as the original waiting room I had found myself in. There were two beds on each side of the room, my girlfriend was with me for support, but I knew she couldn't stay for long, she was allowed about half an hour. There was no one else in the room with us. I wasn't relishing having any company; I wanted to remain on my own with my worries and then in he came. The bed facing mine was occupied alright! But he'd just been terrorising the nursing staff at the end of the corridor. His burgundy dressing gown set the room alight; he glided across the shiny floor in his navy slippers, like a slug with calipers on. Weighing in at 16 stone, he inched up his dressing gown belt and introduced himself. *"Simon's the name, you can see my surname on the end of my bed"* he knew nothing about everything and loved telling me so. We tried to have a quiet moment together, my partner held my hand reassuring me and telling me not to crease my new pyjamas, he was having none of it. We parted with a kiss and rolled our eyes in the direction of our new friend.

I unpacked my bag after watching her leave and felt alone and frightened. I hadn't got my dressing gown out of my bag when he started. *"What's up with you then"?* Before I could get a word out, he was telling me his woes, *"I've got gout, I've got an ulcer, I've got a blood condition, I also have asthma, diabetes and diphtheria, they've done loads of tests but they can't put it right, I know more about this than the doctors and nurses, this is my 27th time I've been in here and they're still no nearer to sorting me out."* I looked at his big round eyes and at the egg yoke on his chin and spoke my first loving words to my new room mate*." Shouldn't you be dead "?* I really needed to be alone. Why had God done this to me? There are millions of sick people in the world that I could have shared a hospital ward with and I was given Simon. I felt vulnerable and sad after my girls parting kiss. God had given me a new friend. Then he started again, he was like a cross between a member of the SS and a customs officer. His interrogation went on. *"So then what you in for"?* His eyes looked longingly all over my bed end for any notes or clues that would feed his curiosity. *"I'm having my testicle removed",* I said quietly *"the snip"?* Came his reply – *"No I've got testicular cancer",* He stuck his lips out, and his eyes darted at an alarming pace all over the room. He looked more worried than me, but somehow I knew he would have all the answers. Suddenly his eyes stopped and he stared right into me, he looked like he was blowing an invisible whistle. *"You'll be fine, it's nothing, a mate of mine had both off and he's sound.* Another lecture was about to start. *"I'll tell you what it is about knackers, you don't need 'em you know, do you heck, you can live a full life without them".* I stared at him as he walked around the room as he engaged his new shit scared audience.*" If I could have mine off I would"* what is this man on I thought. *"Nurse"* he shouted, *"nurse"* she didn't come so he pulled his alarm cord, and then pressed his buzzer, until she responded. *"Now then Sarah, can I have a cup of tea and you better get the new lad one as well. I've* just been telling him he's going to be fine". She rolled her eyes in my direction, she didn't have to speak, and we both knew what a character we were dealing with. He'd been in there a week before I arrived and must have terrorised the poor souls with his demands. She came over and asked if I wanted a cup of tea, *"don't worry sweetheart"* she said, *"you'll get used to him"* I suddenly felt a bit better. *"He's having his testicle off Sarah"* bellowed across the ward *"Yes I'm well aware of that Simon",* came her reply in a quiet but stern voice. *"Which are you having off then"* he said, by now flicking through my bag, checking my things, *"slippers"* and he nods *"paper",* and he nods again. *"Have you brought anything to eat?"* I advised him I was not allowed to eat after 6pm that night. *"Oh flaming Nora, I'm starving. Nurse"* he screamed in my ear – *"you'd better bring us a butty, bring this lad one, we can celebrate losing his ball"* By now there were notes on the end of my bed and he took great delight in finding out who my doctor was to be *"Oh your having Dr Skutt are you?, I always go under with Dr Sloan, knows what he's doing that one. Very few scars left by him you know"*

They had put me in a ward with a madman; eventually he shuffled back to his bed, taking with him, my paper. I was left to put everything back in my bag. He crawled onto his bed, breathing heavily and dragged himself up until he was propped up and steady enough to read my paper from cover to cover.

I got it back some three hours later after he had kindly filled in the crossword and word search for me, before crying out *"Crap, there's nothing in it"* I then got changed into my crisp new pyjamas.

I sat upright in bed trying not to attract his attention, too late, *"we've two other people coming in today"* he shouts. *"Don't you worry, leave it to me pal I will find out what's going on".* What's going on I thought, he was clearly in his own world, he seemed to love it in here, I'm sure I've read articles about people who admit themselves into hospital when there's nothing really wrong with them as he fitted the bill perfectly. I was getting a bit jittery as my operation was to be first thing in the morning and I was trying not to think about what lay ahead. But how could I worry, with my new best mate sat across, smiling at me. *"NURSE"* he shouts again, *"I need a pillow, and he wants one too".* I didn't, but I didn't protest, the poor girl brought me the pillow even though I didn't need one. *"It's my new mate over there",* she understood, *"don't worry, you're getting two new people in today for a bit more company".* She assured me that they couldn't possibly be anything like Simon, *"I don't think you will meet another of his kind if you looked all year".* I was saved from being savaged outright by this medical wonder show when the new arrivals were admitted to fill the other two beds. I tried my best to remain polite to Simon and wanted to warn my new allies who had just arrived what to expect. They arrived within minutes of each other. The guy on my left was very quiet, 35 – 40 years old, balding and kept himself to himself, he seemed to have his own worries. He appeared friendly but only ever nodded, he sat for a while with his wife talking very quietly. Occupying the fourth and final bed was my favourite of all – Alfred he was 75 years young. My first impressions were of a lovely kind old man who had no doubt seen a fare few Simons in his time. He had a kind warm face that was surely to be tested as he was in the next bed to the incredibly ill man mountain. By now Simon was laying on his side telling Alfred the same tale he told me on my arrival. The list of illnesses had grown a little longer and he was now a Black Death survivor.

Alfred looked great for 75 and had a friendly face. He seemed to take a liking to me, and although I didn't know him, he somehow reassured me that everything was going to be ok. I people watched for the next hour as Simon started to tell the entire ward again how ill he was. Alfred was polite and used to give me the odd glance across the room, acknowledging the medical genius in the bed across. The guy in the next bed was just as polite; although he would role over when Simon started discussing how he split an atom at the tender age of three and how all the girls in his class at school camped outside his home, just to get a glimpse of him. There was a time when he had to turn the James Bond role down as he had to look after his elderly Aunt and of how he once slept with 8 girls in one night, each and every one of them climaxing 5 times.

So .....He lived alone and was a virgin!! I had my suspicions that he lived alone or with elderly parents, he didn't appear to have a girlfriend and no one seemed to visit him. He was probably very lonely underneath his cheek. I grew to like him, but would never tell him that.

He entertained me with his blunt cheek and know it all attitude but he was harmless. Everyone, including the staff knew that he was crying out to be loved so we all just put up with his behaviour. He grew on me and he made the long days seem shorter.

There would be 10 minutes peace and quiet then he would start a discussion about my testicle *"he's having his bollock off aren't you?"* It was his way of trying to make a conversation with the guy in the next bed to me. *"He's got cancer, got to have his bollock off, rather him than me. Mind you a mate of mine had them both off and he's fine."* No one was interested. The bloke in the next bed, cranked his head off the pillow, gave me a raised eyebrow, and replied *"You couldn't shout that any louder could you, I don't think they heard you in Ward 10!"*

Alfred broke the ice, *"what do you do for a living lad"* he called over. *"I work in travel"* he seemed genuinely interested. We had a bit of a chat and he asked me about sport. I told him I played open age football and he invited me to sit on the end of his bed as he had a tale to tell

"When I was a lad about 20ish I played rugby for a team, rugby union, it's going back a while I know, but they were good days back then. Our captain of the team had a stammer and he really struggled with his speech. We were playing away and turned up at this ground to play this team and low and behold their captain also had a bad stammer. He suffered just the same. As the two teams warmed up before the game, the captains met up in the middle with the referee to toss for kick off. They shook hands and then all hell broke loose, when their captain tried to speak but stuttered our captain remained silent. Then when our boy spoke up the other bloke thought he was poking fun at him, so he cracked him, so he then cracked him back and then both teams fired into each

other. Before a ball had been kicked we were fighting all over the pitch. The referee couldn't believe it. Anyway the fighting finally stopped and we had a good hard game, there were broken noses and cut lips. Back in the pub after the game, both teams laughed like buggery at what had started from the two stammering captains. These two remained friends for years. I don't think they ever phoned each other though; they wouldn't have been able to afford the phone bill."

Alfred was great company. It was a tale I have told on many occasions and one that tickled me, Alfred had become my friend in the hospital. He was a dry old man with a good sense of humour. *"You'll be fine son"* I remember him saying with a wink *"trust me",* and I did.

As the ward became quiet on the evening prior to my operation, I lay in my bed staring at the ceiling wondering what lay ahead. I was trying to be normal, but one thought kept entering my head. From tomorrow I will only have one testicle, what kind of a man will I be? My situation had started to sink in, hiding feelings might seem like good therapy, but they have a way of coming out at you when you're at your most vulnerable. It was very quiet on the ward, apart from the odd burst from Simon's arse across and his regular attempt at annoying the staff. As the other two snored in unison, I imagined the real Simon collected his thoughts at this time of day, and wondered if he had regrets about his behaviour. Then as If by magic, another one of his farts would rip out and disturb my thoughts.

Had I taken things for granted, my comfy bed, my partner, my friends, my home, and would I wake up from the anaesthetic? I had heard stories and read things in magazines. I wasn't looking forward to having my testicle removed. I wanted to cry, but for some reason couldn't, be strong I kept telling myself. The thought of getting the cancer out of my body helped in a strange way. I tried to concentrate on looking forward to having a beer with the lads and playing football again. I even thought about how I would change my ways, be less of a doormat and concentrate on the things in life I have always wanted to do and never quite got round to doing. I decided that when I was better, then it struck me again that I didn't even feel ill. The funny thing is, although I had testicular cancer I didn't look or feel ill. I was lucky, they had caught it early. The treatment makes you ill, no wonder I was confused. I felt perfectly well and wondered if all of this was really necessary? What if they had made a mistake? Eventually I drifted off to sleep and was gently serenaded by Simon's bodily functions as he slept. He is the only man I have ever met who made as much noise in his sleep, as he did when he was awake.

I wasn't allowed any breakfast in the morning. I've always had a great appetite and breakfast was my favourite. Not today though. Simon was revitalised and ready to belittle me in front of whoever was listening; he was on fine early morning form. His words touched my soul and clattered my hunger pangs as he shouted at the nurses for his own breakfast, farted and looked across at me. *"You wont get ought today mate, you don't you know, coz they're taking your bollock off"*, followed by a large cackle of laughter. I lay silent, looking up at the cracked paint on the ceiling, praying for his colostomy bag to explode. What a lovely man, 07:55 am on the clock and he's off with the first insult of the day. Then the next one came across*." By tea time tonight they'll be 7 knackers in this room"* he laughs out loud again*, "Don't forget the talking prick in your bed"* came the reply from the guy at the side of me.

He winked and rolled over again to face the other way. Alfred was now awake and chuckled away to himself. Simon proceeded to dissect his breakfast and shout across to see if I fancied sniffing his sausage. Was this bloke for real? Unfortunately for me he was. He entertained himself through the meal and laughed between mouthfuls. *"Do you want this button mushroom" you can shove it down your Y fronts tonight"* and again he howled to the ward. Alfred then reminded him of his manners and advised him to eat his breakfast before it went cold, and asked him if he could try and make a bit more noise with his next mouthful. He looked puzzled but it didn't stop him clearing the tray in record time.

My operation was getting nearer and I had almost forgotten about it with all the excitement until a doctor came round to explain the procedure. He asked if I didn't' mind the 7 or 8 student doctors being with him as he went about his business. He reassured me about the operation and discussed how I might feel, once it was all over. He told me how long it might be before I was allowed to go home. *"Have you considered having a false one"?* I was surprised by his question...." *A false one"*, *"what good would that be"?* I asked in all innocence. I didn't want to appear rude or ignorant, but his suggestion seemed to come from nowhere and caught me off guard. *"Some people decide to have a false one put into the scrotum, you really can't tell, its each to their own but it has been said that it can make you feel more complete, more of a man ".* *"Would this enhance my modelling career"?* I asked, he looked startled, the students gave me a smile, *"quite"* he said. *"Do you have a selection I could look at? Have you got any designer ones? Do you have one with the Manchester United badge on"?* He smiled and carried on." *Joking apart, it is an option, just let me know, have a think about it ,even if it's a time after the initial surgery, we can still arrange it. It's a very personal thing".*

I couldn't really take in, what it was he was asking and once again tried to smooth over my ignorance with laughter. Later it did cross my mind, and I could understand why men have it done, but I'd made up my mind. I believed that there had been enough tampering with my area of pleasure to last me a lifetime. It's a snip and it's in, simple as that, he had informed me. As simple as it sounded, I still didn't fancy another operation, even though I hadn't had this one yet.

As he shook my hand to leave, I couldn't resist a pop at Simon *"if you've got any spare false testicles, would you mind inserting half a dozen into the guy in the bed across, the next time he's under the knife"?* He winked and I felt he understood me. He was a lovely man who had a knack of putting people at ease.

Thoughts would pop into my head of how I might cope with only one testicle. How will I manage when I have stopped the jokes and I'm sat alone, will I be a lesser man? What If in the future my relationship brakes down? How would I start again with part of me missing? If it came to it, what girl in her right mind would want a man with one ball?

Back in secondary school one boy had been picked on. A rumour had started how he only had one ball. I remember laughing and joining in without really thinking of how he might have felt. It was irrelevant whether it was true or not, as kids we were so cruel, the shit had stuck and he carried this, all the way through until we left at 16. I was now about to be him. I would have to start again, with one ball, what if my relationship crumbles under this strain.

He was a boy and just shrugged his shoulders and laughed it off, but I was a man and boy was I frightened.

I confided in a friend not long after as we sat and had a pint. *"Listen"* he said *"Any girl that didn't want a man, because he had a testicle missing was not worth knowing at all".* He was right. He then got up out of his seat and picked the two empty pint glasses up to buy the round. He winked to reassure me. As he turned he bent over in his new denim mini skirt and 5 of his balls slipped out of his leather thong, I felt quite normal...........

I was still quite worried that I might be viewed as a somewhat lesser human being or a lesser man. I suppose that I just got on with it....I had to. I never did get the false one. It's a very personal thing, the doctor was right, I've come to terms with having one and it is a beauty and to tell you the truth I can hardly tell. I'm hoping tight stretch jeans never make a comeback. Mind you, I can always slip a sock in if it's that obvious. Testicular cancer does not make anyone a lesser man, negative thoughts have crossed my mind, but as you get on with it, you just seem to get used to it. It's what's inside that matters and I'm not talking Y fronts here

Chapter 30

NO GOING BACK, LEFTY WENT OFF TO THE Y FRONTS IN THE SKY

There was no going back now as I'd just had my pre-med, my partner had been to visit and was my rock. I could tell though that she was feeling the strain. Throughout her visit she had gone on about who had been on the phone, people I hadn't spoken to for years. As she got up to leave before my operation I offered her one last chance to rub the testicle for luck and hold him for one last time. She looked at me on the bed and her stare could have cracked glass."*I'll give it a miss, besides I've got a couple of false ones off the Doctor to use as worry beads, and you can have one off me, if you change your mind*" For us it was just as important that we could both still laugh about it. Our humour helped us come to terms with awkward situations. I was wheeled down to the operating table by a nurse that I already knew and we laughed all the way down, that pre-med stuff blows your mind, literally. I've never done LSD but this stuff can't be much different. "*If I don't come out of here you can have my Man United slippers*", I knew her husband was a red. I've never been into drugs but the stuff they gave me warped my mind, I was on cloud 9 as she wheeled me down. "*When I come out I want to be known as Maureen, I will be half man, half women and part cross dresser*". The garbage that came out of my mouth was bewildering. I wish I'd recorded it. They'd be less wars in this world if all the world leaders had a pre med and then sat down to talk. I informed the nurse of what I required should I wake up. "*I want a bouquet of black roses with just one white one for my lost ball at the side of my bed. If the local papers turn up, just do shots from the right until I get used to walking unaided. I'm selling my kilt because if the wind catches me unawares, it could frighten the neighbours*". I was as free as a bird." *Don't wheel me in the wrong way, they might take one of my ears off and I'll have to sell my walkman*". They pushed me into a lift so I wouldn't disturb anyone in the corridor and I was off again." *SECURITY, SECURITY, their taking my knacker off, it's the left one; I've put a plaster over the right one so you know which one to keep. If you leave it at the side of my bed I will collect it on my return*". They couldn't shut me up. "*I'm going to have it glazed and painted and wear it on a chain around my neck.*" I finally shut up as I remembered the kind nurse's face as something sharp was stuck into the back of my hand..............I was out cold and so peace had returned.

Next thing I remember it was the next morning. The porter came in and shook my hand. "*Hey*" he said, "*I just had to come and have a word with you, what a laugh, and how's the testicle, have you had it glazed yet?*" I had no idea who the hell he was and wanted him arrested. He talked to me as if we had grown up together, I was still in my own world but it now felt terrible. My mouth was as dry as a camels ring piece, my eyes looked at his excitable lips moving too fast for my mind to know what the flaming hell he was on about. He held my hand like a brother and I stared at him, my eyes half open, trying to cry out for help but my lips were stuck together as tight as his grip on my hand. I could taste my breath; it would have made a dung beetles fart smell like roses. I carried on staring at him praying for a flash back. It didn't come I was suffering from the affects of the anaesthetic. I must have entertained him big time. He went on "*I just had to come and see you", you really had me chuckling."*

He then called me Zorro. I struggled to speak, so raised my eyebrows to engage with him and to try and tell him that I didn't know what the flaming hell he was on about. .Apparently I'd been going on that I had a Zorro mask and cape under my operating gown and he was instructed to put it on me the moment my ball was removed. On waking I would bounce around the hospital, beam to beam checking that no mistakes were made and people were getting the correct organs removed. I'd just get there in time and whip off the correct bollock with the tip of my sword and the surgeons would thank me. I was apparently a hero but no one knew it was me behind the mask. It was to be our secret. Apparently I would only turn into Zorro after my pre-med, which is a bit strange as I'd only ever been operated on once before, so I couldn't have been that great a super hero. Even so my bullshit had seemed to make my new friend the porter smile and that was good enough for me.

My ranting about Zorro had appeared somewhat flawed, as the porter pointed out to me that I should have had my mask over my mouth in a hospital and not over my eyes. A minor hiccup I explained, as my new friend the porter left he whispered in my ear *"do me a favour, never ever touch LSD,"* with a wink he went on, *"but if you do, make sure you come and find me and I will sit and listen to the tripe that comes out."* With that he was gone................. !!

As I began to focus and wake up, the small sips of tea I was allowed were heaven sent. Life entered my mouth, even though I felt terrible I was beginning to focus on my surroundings. Oh no I had forgotten about Simon, *"Hey up, one knack"*, was his welcome call, *"how you feeling? Have you dropped a bollock.?"* I felt terrible and didn't need this. Thankfully I was allowed home within a few days. Once I was steady on my feet I was given the green light to leave. I wouldn't particularly miss Simon but I would always remember him.

As I arrived home, the realisation hit me. The staples in my stomach yanked on my sanity every time I coughed or caught them on my new pyjamas. I wasn't prepared for the staples in my stomach, I was ignorant to the procedure and thought they would just nip my sack and take my testicle out without much pain. I was wrong; the surgeon operated through my stomach and took the cancerous testicle out that way.

Chapter 31

RECOVERY

As I began my recovery from the operation, friends and family started to phone and visit. Although the operation was a success, the next hurdle was to be the chemotherapy. I slowly but surely got back on my feet and tried to make sense of it all. The aftercare was amazing. A district nurse came and cared for me. She encouraged me with laughter and honesty. *"You're going to be fine",* she said, *"They've done a real job, it's really neat. You'll soon be up and on your feet".*

I began to get calls from the people I knew at work. My immediate senior staff knew why I was off ill, but I had not told the people close that I worked with. It was a personal thing, I asked the manager to just tell them that I had some stomach problems. I didn't fancy the office knowing that I was losing a testicle. It was a big thing for a bloke to admit to anyone. I felt very odd at that time I didn't want to lie, but I didn't wish for it to be common knowledge. As time went on I didn't mind as much, but you have to get it straight in your mind first before you start discussing it with anyone else. I honestly didn't know how I felt. Later in my recovery I found that I would fill up and get very emotional. There were not many tears though, not because I was trying to be tough, but I just didn't know how to cry. I wasn't brought up to cry.

I was now dealing with the realisation of what had happened to me and that it was not someone else. How dare I get this cancer thing! As daft as it might sound I thought I would live forever. I would get angry when I realised that cancer didn't just happen to......other people.. Even though I had seen my mum go through it I just thought that it would never happen to me. The calls became awkward for my partner to deal with as she didn't know what to say to people who worked with me. I was now struggling to discuss it with her, let alone people at work and so had spells of being very quiet.

People at work must have begun to sense that it was something serious, after all within the space of 4 days I had been admitted into hospital, normally you would get a date and wait, with cancer it's different, and you're straight in.

My partner was beginning to feel the strain, the calls she made when I had been diagnosed were coming back to haunt her. People care and try to help, but she must have spoken to loads of people and the cracks were starting to show on her

She was getting fed up of answering the phone to people asking how I was. I started taking the calls and was stumped for the first time when someone asked how I felt. I held the phone in silence for a time then replied *"How am I? I don't know, I've just had a bollock off, I don't know how I am"*. They went on *"Have they stopped the cancer?"* God I thought. Yes its cancer, I had stopped thinking I had cancer.*" I hope so* "I said stuttering a bit like

Alfred's old rugby chums, *"I'm not sure",* I looked over at my partner, my eyes must have said it all, I didn't know what I was supposed to say. It's probably just as bad for the person asking the questions. *"I didn't like to ring"* they said. *"I'd heard second hand, are you going to be ok"?* I stuttered through the call and then took it off the hook. The phone call had made me realise again that cancer was now apart of my own life whether I liked it or not.

The surgeons move that quick with the diagnosis and the surgery that your life can appear to change overnight, one minute your jack the lad, doing normal things, the next you're discussing losing a testicle on the phone. It can take a while to sink in. One of my best friends who had been working away popped round to see me. He hadn't heard of my dilemma at the time. He came in and looked shocked as I explained what had happened *"I thought you were off work with a cold, slumbering around in your pyjamas."* He went white. He stayed for a drink and as I sat on the sofa staring at the floor I could hear my partner in the kitchen explaining to him what had happened. It was beginning to sink in.

I was worried, tired and overwhelmed by peoples concern and words of kindness. I think I had started to take on their worries. I realised that all I was doing was reassuring them, when really I didn't know myself. I heard myself telling people I was going to be fine, but deep down all I really wanted was for someone to tell me that I would be ok. I thought back to mum and how she had looked after me when she had just been diagnosed.

Cancer changes your life in an instant. My whole world was now upside down. This time last week I was happy going about my business, now I've got staples in my stomach a ball missing and worried friends and family.

My friend stayed a while and after he had gone I sat alone downstairs.

I remember looking at our cat Audrey Maud Knapton. I watched him groom himself in his own little world. I thought, *"You don't give a shit do you"*? He scratched his head and looked at me. This animal wouldn't care if I had no balls, fur balls or three balls, he'd still look at me just the same. I'm no different in the cat's eyes, as crazy as it seemed, thinking like this kind of helped. I stroked his head and then hit it with a mallet. Pure therapy, I was beginning to feel better already, thankfully our cat always groomed himself with a crash helmet on. As he sat there scratching and sneezing, blowing his germs all over me, he stuck a paw in the air and popped out a claw in my direction as it continued to lick his balls....this was one smart cat.

I was now at home with plenty of time to think, plenty of time to worry and plenty of time to do nothing. The second I forgot about my staples, I got a quick reminder as I got up quickly or coughed. Gradually I improved and in time was up and down tottering between the bathroom, the kitchen fridge and winding myself up looking for the TV remote. Daytime TV helped to blacken my mood. I started to get some very strange thoughts, it was as if I was trying to speed up my life, I started planning things, we had the smallest garden imaginable, it's that small that we once got some artificial turf from a garden centre to try and grow a lawn, but it was too small to fit a mower into the area. We cut the turf to fit, fed and watered it, and low and behold our mini lawn was born. As the grass started to grow, the neighbour next door couldn't contain himself. *"I've seen it all now"* he said as I was lying on my side cutting the grass with kitchen scissors. He shook his head laughing and went back inside. My life now seemed to be one of planning. It was as if I was frightened of having no future so I felt I had to cram everything into all my days .One day I meticulously planned the layout of the back yard, drew it as technically as I could. I sewed the seeds in my head of how it would look. I'd planned what kind of stone I would get, the flowers, the look and colour scheme, this was never in my nature to do such a thing before. Had my diagnosis changed me? The gardening before was never my thing, It was never a priority with me.

Chapter 32

MONTHS OFF WORK & LOSING IT BIG TIME

It now seemed that I was rushing to do the things I had previously put off. I planned how our front room would look with a brand new 5 foot fish tank in the corner, another passion of mine, I had neglected. As I became more agile I arranged for people to give me lifts to pick up the necessary items for the garden and could not wait to get cracking. It was a very strange time; I felt that I was in a permanent rush. Was I covering my anxiety up with tasks I knew interested me? Maybe it was to take my mind off my worries? I wouldn't accept any help from anyone who wanted to help. I am not a freak I kept telling myself.

People were wonderful and genuine with their intentions to assist, but my patience was wearing thin. My lovely next door neighbour visited one day and insisted that he help out. I was building a small wall in the corner of the garden. I had acquired some garden centre stones to cement together and had my idea on how it would look against the backdrop of flowers and plants I had chosen.

All he wanted was to help, he cared, but I needed and wanted to be on my own, I needed to feel normal.

I was never one for gardening or DIY before being told about the cancer. It was as if the diagnosis had prompted me to prove I could do things. Before cancer entered my own life I wouldn't have bothered either way but, now I was on a mission. My elderly neighbour stood over me and took the bucket of cement out of my hand and proceeded to take control. His intentions were honourable, I had the most amazing respect for him, he was an ex service man with 30 years in the army behind him and a strict disciplinarian. We were an odd couple, I was like the rough squaddie, that needed licking into shape and he was the Sergeant Major that was going to do it. Many times in the past I had bitten my tongue as he barked orders at me to pump up my car tyres, cut my hair, smarten myself up and make an honest woman of my girl. He was my friend and mentor but I needed to do this alone.

The task in hand was not difficult, but I felt he didn't understand how I was feeling. I had brought some bags of compost to lay behind the wall in which I was to plant my creation in and he proceeded to cut open the bags in readiness for taking over the job. I tried to remain calm, but I was starting to fail, within a breath he was on his hands and knees flattening the soil that was already in there with his bare hands. I knew there was a god, for before he had started interfering I'd noticed it being full of cat shit, it was where our cat headed every night when we let it out. I smiled to myself as I watched him flatten the shit soaked soil with his bare hands. He flattened it with the palm of his hands, then wiped his forehead, stood up, admired his work and began to praise himself for his handy work. On any other day I would have warned him about the cat's toilet and what he was messing with. The devil was in me that day as I smirked to myself. He carried on and proceeding to take over the job, I was instructed to get some water for mixing the cement, *"chop chop, we need to crack on"*. He was only trying to help me, but just at that moment I lost it. Like a spoilt child I threw the spade to the ground and stormed into the house. Although it was only a spot of gardening to most, at that time it was a massive thing for me. I think I was trying to prove deep down that I was capable of doing these tasks on my own and that I had every right to remain on this earth doing the things that other people normally do.

Chapter 33

TRIALS

As my treatment for the illness progressed, I became involved in a scheme to keep a tab of how I felt. It was a trial run by the cancer hospital, to get an idea on what kind of things go through patient's minds. Every time I went, I filled in forms and answered questions on a touch screen computer. They wanted to discover the thoughts and feelings behind the illness, my moods, my thoughts, and to see if I was anxious, irritable, angry or upset. The trial was to help them understand. From the very beginning I had come to understand that this type of illness was just as challenging mentally as it was physically.

My poor neighbour had found that out. We soon made up though and I was made to run around the block 46 times with the spade above my head in the pouring rain. I was court-martialled and banned from all leave for 5 years. He told me that he was only trying to help. I knew he genuinely was, but my patience had been stretched to the limit but thankfully it was soon forgotten and we remained friends. I never did tell him though about the cat shit. If he ever interfered again I would smile to myself, It was a kind of therapy. Particularly when he would slate the cat and say" *the best thing you can do with that thing is to have it put down".* He wasn't a cat lover, but I was. I'd stroke him with my mallet and thank him for shitting in the plants.

My moods would go from wanting to take on the world to down right depression. I was snappy and irritable and felt like a victim. As the phone calls became less and less I felt I was on my own, even though everyone I knew had been wonderful. I realised that it was going to be a long road. I wanted to get back to normal, get back to work and to play football again.

Chapter 34

SAVING SPERM

It was to be another 6 weeks before I had my chemotherapy and I was still at home recovering from the surgery. I had spent a long time alone while my partner was at work, thinking about what had happened to me and how I was now fed up to my back teeth with day time TV and cups of tea. I knew the date to have my treatment was approaching and was really not looking forward to chemotherapy. It was then that I was asked if I would like to save my sperm. In short it means giving samples that are stored for later use. This is done if there is damage to your sperm count by the chemotherapy, as it can make you infertile. I was curious and not sure of the procedure and what was expected of me. After discussing it with my girlfriend, I had made my mind up to do it. We didn't have children and hadn't really talked about whether we were going to have any in the future. But now this had made me think about it, especially as there was the possibility that I may end up not being able to have any at all. It became a real issue. I was to be driven to the hospital by my Sergeant Major friend next door along with my partner who came along to support me. The hospital was to advise me of the results of my sperm count, then arrange for me to make more deposits so they could keep them in storage should I require to use them in the future. I was advised to make as many trips as possible before my treatment began. The more sperm the better, as it would give me more chances of fathering a child should the situation arise. What an experience this turned out to be!

Chapter 35

TAKING THE FUN OUT OF MASTURBATING

I couldn't believe I was going to Leeds to masturbate and it was all legal and above board. Between visits I was told to avoid any sexual contact with my partner as this would affect the strength of my sperm count.

At home It was as if she knew, and had taken on a new identity in the house as she swanked about, knowing full well that I couldn't pounce on her, as regularly as before. Well as regular as every March, usually on my birthday or Christmas. It had a strange affect on me, when something is taken away from you, you seem to want it twice as much as you did before.

I would test the water and sit on the sofa in a leather cat suit, waiting for her to come in from work, polishing the crutch with "Mr Sheen". She would respond by dusting the cobwebs off it and spraying me with bromide to kill my urges. I would dance around her, whilst she watched TV.I was like a peacock, teasing, purring and pouting my lips until she got so fed up that she would call the police who would threaten me with arrest or eviction.

I finally got the message and stopped pestering her but then had a vision of struggling to get my 12lb testicle into the car on my next trip to the hospital. I wasn't disappointed as it usually took 5 porters and my elderly neighbour to get me and my testicle out of the car and into the lift. I bought a new wheelbarrow for the next journey to save my neighbours back. It was a good job I didn't have to do this once a month or it would look like I was travelling around on a space hopper.

On my first time I was getting worried on how I might perform and what was the exact procedure. In the car on the way there my mind was racing, I began to feel the pressure. I tried to admire the scenery out of the window but my bulge restricted the view, it was as if an airbag had gone off by mistake in the back of the car. When we stopped in traffic, passers by would stare in to try to get the driver's attention. One old lady put her head through the open window and asked how much he wanted for the dinghy in the back. I felt like a survivor on a sunken ship, clinging to the side of a life raft.

Like any red blooded male that enjoyed the odd tickle with his tackle, I usually did it alone and in private. This situation I was now in was very different and seemed so much more clinical, somehow the fun had been taken out of it.

I felt like a performing seal, I was concerned where I would have to do it and prayed that I would not be in a line with other men in the same position as me, hoping I would be left alone. It seemed crazy; I had been given the green light to play with myself.

We arrived at the clinic and I was asked to wait while a nurse attended to me. I was a little apprehensive as it's a very personal thing. After a 10 minute wait I was greeted by a male nurse, he took myself and my girlfriend into a side room and began to explain. I wasn't bothered that she was with me; he did ask though if it was ok for her to attend. Not a problem I thought, but did I mean it?

He began to explain *"Today if you can produce a sperm sample for us we can work out your sperm count and tell you next week when you come back what level it's at"*. What level's it at? He continued and repeated what he had just said, *"today I need you to produce a sample and next week when you come back, you can do me another one."* *"Hang on a minute"* I interrupted, *"You want me to come back next week and do it all again"* my mind was racing, my erection fading.

"Yes, we need you to produce as much of your sperm as possible". He explained that it would be beneficial for me and my partner in the future should the chemotherapy damage my sperm count and affect our chances of conceiving. I had expected to drop in today, produce once and once only and that would be it. From what I could gather he was expecting me to come back time and time again. He went on, *"before you get your date for chemotherapy, you need to come as many times as possible, no pun intended"* he said, as he moved his head closer to mine across the table. Now as embarrassed as I was, this man put me at ease and I took an instant liking to him. I got the impression he liked me too. He had a sense of fun and what a job he had!

I liked his chin beard that had a blue bead attached to the end of it. I liked his style; he had a fun like sparkle in his eyes. I remarked to my partner about the colour of his clogs when he first greeted us, one red, and one yellow. This guy didn't care; he was as cool as a cucumber as we discussed my 46 inch marrow, we both enjoyed the banter and could sense each others easy going attitude.

Looking deep into my eyes and leaning forward across the table he had compassion in his voice. *"Mr Turner, if you and your lovely lady are to increase your chances of having children, then you will have to put the work in".* *"And what hourly rate will I be on?"* I enquired. He rolled his eyes; he knew he could get away with being himself with us and we sensed he enjoyed our company and his job. *"Now the choice is obviously up to you and your lovely girl. I'm here to help, though not literally mind".* *"I should think not",* I said. *"It's as simple as that, the more you produce, before chemo, the more we can store, should you need it in the future for IVF etc. You will probably receive your treatment date soon. You should have around two weeks to come and see me and fill up some jars with your manly prowess".*

I enquired about the size of the jars, hoping they weren't like beer barrels. *"Not very big, I'm sure you won't have any problems, a fine boy like you",* smiling at my girl and turning his head at speed to make his point. *"I will be with you all the way, to help you as I can see that's what you're worried about!"* He tried to reassure me again *"Don't worry you'll be on your own at the moment or moments of truth, there's no perks in this job".* We all laughed. So there it was, he had explained it in sample, sorry simple terms. I could make as many visits as I wished in the time I had before my chemotherapy started. It was like my first bank account, the more I produce, the more they save, and the better the chance of us starting a family in the future.

"Let's get my little wrigglers wriggling then" I thought I would only be going once and getting it over with, but this guy put me at ease, he knew what he was doing. He

knew how to deal with people, and as easy going as I was, masturbating to a timescale was very different to doing it for fun hiding in the cellar, or the linen basket in next door's bathroom.

I had been told in my original letter to abstain from having sex up to 3 days before this visit so that my little wrigglers would be bouncing about, ready to rock and roll so that this would give a clearer reading of my sperm count. I had been as good as my word and had not interfered with myself or the girlfriend for the last three days. *"Should I take up knitting if I get the urge"* I asked her, *"yes, you can do me a scarf and a pair of bright orange mittens"* she replied. I wish I hadn't asked.

So here I was about to enter the unknown and masturbate with another man. *"What if I can't perform"* I asked, *"I'm not a robot you know"*. *"Oh I'm sure you will perform, just let your imagination run wild! And anyway I will be there to help in anyway I can"*. My partner was given a cup of tea with 12 brandies in while I set off with him, hand in hand. I turned and looked at her, it felt a bit like betrayal, does she mind? What's she thinking? What would I think if it was the other way round? Oh sod it; I'll just enjoy it while I have permission. I splashed my ball with aftershave and skipped down the corridor. The excitement definitely wasn't the same as sneaking about at home when she had the washer on and she couldn't hear me shouting out as I lost myself.

We entered yet another clinical looking room with a bed and a sink, a bed I thought, how long is this going to take as he handed me a folder. *"That's for you"*, I looked at it and now I was feeling nervous *"is this my insurance?"* He instructed me to open it. *"It's got adult literature in, these magazines should help to start you off."*

I asked him for a pen, *"a pen"?* He looked startled *"The crossword"* he laughed, and handed me a paper bag and a plastic sample bottle that was as wide as a 10 pence piece. I looked at the size of it and looked back at him, *"what"?* He said, *"how am I going to fit it in there, I've got over three days in me you know and besides it's hardly wide enough"* His eyes widened *" its all about control, just control yourself,".* he could see the funny side in his job and he was great fun.

As he turned to leave I held out my arms as if wanting to cuddle him. He looked startled,*" Can we have some heavy petting before I get going please?"*

There was laughter in his voice,*" be off with you".* Just as the door was closing, I peeped through the small gap. *"How long do I stay in here for*?" He shouted back down the corridor *"take your time enjoy yourself, but be warned I finish at 4 o'clock and I'm going out tonight, Just fill the container, clean yourself up, put it in the bag and bring it to me in reception".* I wasn't letting him go without a fight. *"Have you got a couple of carrier bags? You shouldn't underestimate me I was a bit of a gigolo in my youth".* The clicking of his clogs got fainter until it faded into the distance and he was gone. Then a thought struck me, what if I go straight out within a couple of minutes, he's going to think I'm a right wimp. How long should all this take?

With my new friend gone I was now alone with my jar and folder. What if it's a wind up? And it's a copy of farmers weekly or horse and hound.

I won't go into detail but the next 7 hours were bliss. The magazines now resembled Black Beards treasure map. They had well and truly been read from back to front and back again, with of cause the odd peep at the pictures. The crosswords were complete and I was ready to face the world again, refreshed, 3 stone lighter and in love with another 12 women.

I saw the funny side, but it was a strange and most essential experience for me. It was an experience I am glad I went through as I was not sure of the future or if I would be able to father children, it was a time of reassurance in a time of doubt and worry. My friend the caring Clog man later explained that they would keep my sperm for 10 years, frozen and ready to use, should we decide the time is right.

My loving sample was studied and I was shocked to find out that my sperm were slow swimmers, I was most put out as my male ego kicked in and I tried to blame it on the pressure I was put under in the cold grey room and on my disliking of his clogs. I attended a further 4 times and kept up my relationships with the girls in the magazines, each time it got harder and harder to say my goodbyes. One day on the way home in the car a fit of jealousy came over me as I had visions of the clog man lending my magazine to other men. These were my girls and I was struggling to come to terms with sharing. A crack to the side of my head from the other half soon brought me back down to earth, as she reminded me who I belonged to.

I then started to worry that maybe I would become addicted to climaxing in small containers and would eventually work my way through all her Tupperware set. Would I become a swimming coach to try and encourage my little wriggles to speed up? I'd climax in a pink sandwich box whilst I coached them as they jumped into the tub. I'd start wearing a swimming cap and shout *"faster, faster"* at the top of my voice to encourage them. Would my girlfriend become curious about the strange noises coming from the bathroom? What If I started covering myself in lard like the channel swimmers? What If I found myself leaning over the bath with my goggles, lard and Speedos, waiting for the gun to go off as I concentrated my aim in the direction of her favourite cake box? Would this affect our sex life? Maybe the only way I could get excited with her, would be to wear a tight blue swimming cap emblazoned with the hospitals logo.

My mind raced with scenarios of my beloved telling me off for running around the bed in my waders and armbands. I was struggling to sleep with my armbands on anyway and the 6 foot inflatable killer whale between us was starting to irritate her. I'd worked it out; I would have around 10 thousand little wrigglers stored in a deep freeze in the hospital. How could we possibly think of names for all of them, and birthdays would be a nightmare!! The poor postman would break his back on Father's Day. What, if in time I received letters from the hospital for maintenance? It could financially break us.

My sperm were to be stored for 10 years in total and I would receive information on how they were doing at school. Back down on planet earth...and to be serious for a second, I would receive a letter from the hospital asking if I wanted to keep them stored every so often or would I mind letting them perish. I always said yes to keep them as at the back of my mind I never really knew what might happen.

I would have to sign a form to say yes or no and this happened many times over the years after my treatment.

Chapter 36

THE NURSES AND STAFF

All the staff especially the doctors and nurses were wonderful. They help to put you at ease, I'm sure not everyone will have the same warped outlook on life as yours truly but they really do help. They have the magical ability; they are true carer's and can put people at ease in the most personal and emotional of times. They are so adaptable to people and their needs. They care for the young, the old, the frightened, the damned right rude and the likes of me, the frightened lunatics of this world who try to hide behind a mask of humour.

We all cry out in our own way which is when they shine their richness in our direction. My partner at the time was a nurse; her very words echoed this as we sat in the ward in the early frightening days of my diagnosis. We looked on as they worked their magic in front of prying eyes. She said *"the care that these nurses give is second to none; there is a quality to their work. It is as if they are not only working, but giving much of themselves at the same time"*. Her words were delivered in a slow and serious fashion; there was no expression on her face.

I knew she meant every word. What she said hit home and so I was comforted, I knew I was in good hands, wherever this journey took me.

Throughout my journey, through the very personal trauma of testicular cancer, I have been moved by how these wonderful people just get on with it. The whole cancer experience is made so much easier by these remarkable people. Doctor's, nurses and staff who are under so much pressure, but shine and become friends to people who need them.

Chapter 37

My Very Short Career in Nursing

I would like to refer to a conversation I had with my better half. I mentioned that I may contemplate working in this field of work, maybe not as a nurse, but in some capacity as a carer, perhaps looking after the elderly. My timing couldn't have been any worse. For this was after a 12 hour shift she had just completed in the nursing home, where she worked at the time. She was clearly on a high, still in her uniform and dusting everything in sight as the adrenalin was clearly still pumping through her veins after a pretty stressful and chaotic shift. Her words shook me but had us both laughing out loud.

She stared into me with that serious look that any man might recognise when his partner is in serious mode. *"You a carer, don't make me laugh?* As she ran the duster over the top of the TV she continued with her attack *"You struggle wiping your own arse, let alone a total stranger. You wouldn't last a minute, the first smell of shit and you would be off like a shot"*

With that most caring comment, my career in nursing came to an abrupt end.

Chapter 38

CHEMO

With my little wriggles tucked up for the next 10 years I had the reassurance that if the chemotherapy did alter my chance of starting a family, I had these as backup. My girl felt the same as we'd discussed the situation at length. My swimming cap, inflatable killer whale, armbands and her Tupperware set had been banished from the house as it was beginning to put a strain on our relationship.

My next trip into the unknown was to be the treatment that fights the cancer – in my case chemotherapy. The hospital had decided I should have a large dose of chemo rather than radiotherapy; these are the two treatments that fight cancer. I was given my date for the chemo and was informed of the after effect, and what chemotherapy does to the body, how it affects and fights the cancer.

The tricky bit for me was that I didn't feel ill at all, yes I'd had a dull ache, yes I'd had my testicle removed and although the surgery, like any other I imagine, has its own pain, apart from this I felt absolutely fine. It crossed my mind that

It wasn't necessary. However I had learned to trust in these people who clearly knew best. They know what they are doing, and I was aware that research is constantly ongoing to fight cancer.

My partner and neighbour again took me to the hospital for my chemotherapy. I was apprehensive and frightened. As I arrived I felt very humble, and although I had caring people around me, once again felt alone. A needle that allowed the chemo to enter my body was attached to the back of my hand. The pain in my hand got worse the longer I stayed attached to the drip that pumped the chemicals into me. Slowly it worked its way into my bloodstream. The pain in the back of my hand got the better of me and I yearned to rip it out.

As my girl and neighbour left for a coffee, I sat alone attached to the machine – oh how sorry I felt for myself – why me –it was now serious. I've lost a testicle and have had to give my sperm for storing & freezing, and now I'm attached to a drip pumping chemicals into me when I don't even feel ill. The ache was getting worse as I began to feel even sorrier for myself. I stared at the needle in my arm and looked at the bag of chemicals hanging above to the side. I knew that the clear liquid was slowly going to make me ill. Anger began to consume me.

Luckily it didn't last, as my eyes caught a glimpse of someone in the bed at the end of the ward. He looked younger than me, about 25 years old and he too was attached to the same type of machine. The difference between him and me was that I still had all my hair. I felt a total arse. I had been complaining and feeling sorry for myself, when all along this man had been attached to his own machine which was clearly not for the first time. His young face had a settled look. We were the only two people in the ward and we were sharing the same experience. This was chemo area. This is where they make you better; this is where they save lives, this is where they keep families together. We both nodded, he was too far away to speak to. I would have had to shout to communicate with him, but we both had a connection, this was my first encounter with chemotherapy. He'd lost all his hair and he was still attached to a machine, having even more of this stuff pumped into him.

I felt so incredibly fortunate that I'd been told I should only require one large dose and that it wouldn't affect my life. I thought about him and about how lucky I really was. This guy knew what it was going to do to him as he'd had it before. I felt like a fraud and a fool. There I was whinging to myself and all along there are people a lot worse off than me. I stared, not at him, but straight forward, my mind was blank, I'd even forgotten about the pain in my hand. Even though I had read all the leaflets and had been warned by the doctors and nurses of what to expect, I didn't really know what it would do to me. This man knew, and still he sat there on his drip, he sat there like a warrior before the assault. God knows what went through his head. Maybe I was at an advantage as I was ignorant as to what these chemicals were going to do to me. I knew that it killed the bad cells as well as the good cells, the red and the white, the same colours of my favourite football team. Oh how I wished I was there watching them, anywhere but here.

The man across the room sat there very still and calm waiting for every drip to kick in, knowing what was coming. He was a fine looking man; he made me feel very humble in his presence. I was on the drip until the last drop of chemo made its way into my body. Soon I was on my way home, apart from the ache where the needle had been in my arm, I felt absolutely fine. I had been advised though that the treatment would make me ill. I left with half a dozen grey cardboard hats, ready for my sickness bouts, these were to be my companion for the next few days.

Chapter 39

WHAT WAS HAPPENING TO ME?

My usual good appetite had gone; I couldn't face food of any sort. I spent that evening laying on the settee waiting for the medication to kick in. How do you prepare for knowing your going to be ill? I knew the chemo was going to help me, even though I was advised it wouldn't feel like it at the time. Waiting to be sick when you feel fine, I was a little tired; it was like waiting for a hurricane to hit. The shutters were up and I'd boarded up my belongings waiting for the storm. My grey cardboard trilbies that I had been issued with to vomit into were my sandbags, my boarding pass out of this madness and my journey's companion.

I began to feel very weary and tired. I had my first wave of sickness that evening, and my poor partner must have been sick of hearing me throw up. I hadn't eaten but I was still vomiting. My thoughts went back to the young man in the chemo ward. He gave me strength, even though I didn't know him, I knew I wasn't alone. I wasn't the only person feeling bad today. No doubt his hurricane had hit and he was in the eye of his own storm. I wondered if he thought of me.

Strangely, knowing that he had had it before gave me an inner strength. The very fact that he'd had chemo time and time again, made me realise that it must be doing something good or why would he keep going through with it. I walked up to bed weary from the day's events, didn't sleep much, my trilby was on hurricane watch at the side of my bed. The next day as I woke, I knew I was in the eye of the storm. I was vomiting from the moment I awoke. My mouth tasted like a scrap yard, I felt like I had metal Mickey's teeth in. Now I've never tasted any form of metal, but this is how I imagined it would be. I felt I was turning into a radiator. As the day progressed I felt weaker and weaker. The next few days were the worst. You feel like you've just run the London Marathon with Jimmy Saville on your back. No energy, no appetite, no energy to vomit with. The next few days were a blur. I just lay on the settee curled in a ball, lifeless. My girlfriend would stroke my hair and face, I had no energy. The treatment robs you of your good cells and you feel so very tired.

We'd been instructed not to have visitors as at this time I was susceptible to picking up infections. My immune system was very low. So I had no visitors, as anyone with a common cold could spark a case of pneumonia. I could hear the phone going between bouts of sleep followed by even more sickness. I had to keep telling myself it was doing me good, fighting any remaining cancer cells that occupied my body. I was irritable, but had no energy to be irritable; I lay there like a wounded animal. Animals tend to lick their wounds, I didn't try, for one I had no energy and two I couldn't bend that far down.

Chapter 40

The Cat's Revenge in the Eye of My Storm

I lay motionless on the settee, my face on a cushion staring ahead in the direction of that bloody cat. For years it had felt like a second class citizen, frequently getting chucked out by yours truly, into the cold night from in front of the warm cosy fire. His time for revenge had arrived and his timing was perfect. I lay there close enough to smell his beautiful tuna fish breath and felt wasted. I had no choice but to watch him licking his balls in front of the fire. He turned until his rear end was in perfect symmetry with my dead eyes; he turned then shuffled and then sat with both of his back legs sticking out propped up by its front two. He might as well have been sat in a deckchair on the front in Margate; the only thing missing was a pale blue handbag hanging off his paw and a kiss me quick hat.

As he faced me, he began licking his belly, my mind was blank as I watched, waiting for my next sickness bout. He then nuzzled his teeth deep into his thick fur, he may have been a Tom Cat with a girls name ,but he was most certainly a cats cat. The greatest of all insults was then thrust upon me, he then suddenly stopped and stared, I'm sure he winked. Then with slow and deliberate strokes of his rough tongue, began to groom the finest pair of fur genitalia this side of the Yorkshire Pennines. Each stroke was aimed at me, each and every lick of his nuts was for me, now call me insane but I know cats are prone to a six sense and this little fellow knew exactly what he was doing. That cat knew what I'd had done. He was in my direct eye line and I didn't have the energy to look away. He had got me, hook line and sinker lick lick, lick, look up at me, lick, lick, lick, look at me again. It was as if he was rubbing it in that he had a pair of balls to lick and was enjoying the moment. It was as if he knew I was vulnerable and wasn't going anywhere, it was pay back time.

I hadn't the energy to laugh; I was well and truly beaten. After his balls had been spotlessly cleaned, up he got, and sniffed my face; this little shit knew what he was doing. I'd had girlfriends in the past with bad breath, but nothing quite like this. To finish me off, he jumped up and sat on me. Now he either knew I wouldn't push him off or he knew I was in a bad way and wanted to care for me. He knew he wasn't allowed on the settee, but took his chance. We had a love hate relationship.

This cat had a great sense of humour and knew how to take the piss. I had no energy to push him off, and no energy to shout for my partner, so he just sat there. I moved my face the best I could as it sniffed all around me, if only I had my mallet. He eventually jumped down and got comfy in front of the fire. Twenty minutes later and he walked to the door, opened it, pointed its paw into the dark night and beckoned me to leave.

It reminded me of the time I lived at home with my mum when she shouted me into the kitchen to tell me that Tiffin our cat at the time, was dancing across the floor. *"She's not dancing Mum; she's scratching her arse on your lino".* Her piles had been bothering her again. On that... feline Fred Astaire was being kicked out of the front door with mum shouting obscenities in the cat's direction. *"You dirty little ...."* *"Put some pepper down mum that will stop her".* She was beside herself as she explained she'd been watching her go from one end of the kitchen to the other, dragging her fur arse across the floor, mum had encouraged her, clapping her hands in glee as she witnesses the dancing cat. She couldn't believe her eyes at such a talent. Before the kettle had boiled to calm her nerves the mop and bucket were out clearing up its little routine.

I was now getting weaker and weaker, no energy to vomit, I couldn't even drag myself to the bathroom. How I hold my hands up to the people that have countless sessions of chemo. My mouth just got even more metallic, our cat was now bored of abusing me and I felt weaker than ever.

My partner then had to go back to work and so I battled with my next obstacle... constipation. On this occasion the chemo had robbed me of the one thing that I had always relied on, my sense of humour. I had no energy as I sat on the lavatory waiting for nature to work its magic. For two long hours I sat and I tried, but it was no use I knew my body needed to function in the way we all do, but the chemicals had won once again. With no energy to assist me, I was beaten. I felt crushed; it was as if the whole journey I was on had suddenly come down to this one moment. The hidden torment had surfaced, the brave face that I had put on for my friends and family had faded. I had begun to crumble. I couldn't take any more and I slid to the floor. I laid there with nothing left. I was beaten; I curled up and lay there motionless. The tears came......I wept as I felt helpless.

I was alone in the house with no energy to do the most basic of tasks. I stayed there for what seemed hours, I was a pathetic figure, I had let my barriers down and I felt that this thing had me beaten. My energy and dignity taken away by the very chemicals that was supposed to help me. I lay on the floor and wept.

Constipation was one thing I had not envisaged. I'd been on the bathroom floor for what must have been hours, when my partner found me as she came in from work. It was as if all my life source and dignity had been drained from me. Now I really did feel like I was ill. They had been so right; the chemotherapy had wiped me out. It takes time for your good cells to start producing again. Once this process starts, in time you will be able to do more, when you start to feel better. By now I was at my lowest ebb. My partner helped me onto our bed while I rested. She was a nurse and helped me with a suppository. Within half an hour I felt I was passing a 12 foot oak table and 6 matching chairs. I had never felt so undignified and helpless. Things surely couldn't' get any worse could they? Looking back I realised that that afternoon was by far my lowest moment along with the shock of my original diagnosis. I rested on the bed for the best part of the day, staring at the ceiling feeling empty. I then understood why in the clinical trial I was involved in they asked me questions about my feelings and emotions. I felt like I'd been smacked in the face by a 7 stone cod, like a boxer on the ropes knowing he's getting a good hiding but there's nothing he can do about it. How it would be easier to fall to the canvas and give in, but something keeps him standing there against the ropes. He feels the first couple of punches but the rest that are raining down on him are not registering; he's just going through the motions of being battered.

Chapter 41

I Have a Love Rival.......
The Vacuum Cleaner!

As I lay on the bed, feeling sorry for myself the sound of the Hoover downstairs broke my chain of thought. I had always got annoyed at the sound of someone vacuuming; I know it's a necessity in most homes, but my partner had a wonderful relationship with hers and if I had a love rival it was certainly the vacuum cleaner. It was as if they had a wonderful bond, one that I could not break. Each seemed obsessed with the other. I would ponder how in the 20th century man could set foot on the moon, learn to fly, and invent the Television, but still every vacuum I had ever heard, sounded like a £12 second hand banger struggling up a steep hill. Surely someone could make one that was silent.

With more time to think about things, I began to question why when she was doing the carpet, how come she was always doing the bit I was standing on and how annoying it was when she would ram it into my ankles as I sat trying to read the paper. It was as if the two of them were enjoying annoying me. She would vacuum up at any opportunity and I hated how it broke my chain of thought and killed the silence. I wouldn't have bothered at this point in my life if she'd have pushed the vacuum up and down my body whilst I lay there. I hadn't given up but my body appeared to have done because of the treatment – and at that moment in time I didn't seem to care less. She could have rolled me over, dusted me, stuck a daffodil up my backside, sprayed me with polish and laid me on the windowsill, for all to see and It wouldn't have bothered me. Visions of coming out of my trance and finding myself staring out from the middle of the vacuum bag kept coming to the forefront of my mind.

It was hard for my partner; it must have been, as she could see that I didn't appear to have any fight left in me. As jealous as I was about her relationship with the vacuum cleaner I knew she was losing herself in her chores, and doing the usual things like offering me drinks, drinks I really needed but didn't want. In my self pity it was easy to forget how the people who cared about me were feeling and what thoughts they were experiencing. The house was immaculately clean, so clean in fact, that I suspected her and the vacuum were trying to start a family, they had spent that much time together. It was important for her to stay strong at this point, not just for me but for her own sanity. I must have been a swine to live with. She'd noticed I hadn't been washing, my dignity fading, my hair greasy and my moods erratic. At times I would look for someone to blame, maybe the smokers' I knew, for I had never smoked and I felt justified in my anger toward them or anyone.

The metal taste in my mouth was getting worse and my energy levels were depleting. I had no company while she was out at work, but to be honest I wouldn't have noticed if a band of Cossacks came out of the fireplace on horseback and started pillaging the house.

The trial at hospital asked me many questions, covering emotions, moods and fears. On my regular visits I would again take time to fill in questionnaires and answer questions on a touch screen computer about how I felt and if I had any pain or discomfort. The research would help other people and it was comforting having an outlet for my mixed up emotions and worries. They were the type of questions no one at home, friends or family were asking, no one was at fault for not asking me anything, it just didn't seem like the done thing.

The screen probed away!!

1. What kind of thoughts are you having? ... English ones!
2. Are you irritable? .... No I'm flaming not!
3. Do you have feelings of anger? .... No...now sod off!
4. Do you have negative feelings? ...... No, but do you own a gun? What percentages of your thoughts are angry? ....None but I'm f**** furious
5. Do you wish to talk about how you feel? ...... No. but Did I ever tell you about

****

It was as if the screen knew me, no one at home had asked me about my inner feelings, and no one had asked me if I felt a lesser man, no one had enquired if I had feelings of anger or frustration. My emotions were being examined on the screen and boy did it help. Things started to make sense. Yes I feel like I want to scream. Yes I feel like I want to cry. Yes there are times when I don't want to talk about how I feel. Yes there are times when I feel like a freak. Yes there are times when I wish it had never happened to me or to my family. My mood swings really surprised me. One minute I was agitated and bitter, the next, I was like Gandhi stroking a leaf, smiling from ear to ear. I was angry and emotional, and then I could suddenly feel exceptionally happy at being alive.

The questions from the trial made me realise I was normal, that maybe it must be right to feel this way. Why would they ask me if it wasn't? I'd always hidden behind my humour, but cracks were appearing, you can only wear a mask for so long without it slipping. Humour helps as laughing made me feel good, but someone constantly laughing would eventually get locked up. I didn't want to turn into one of those people that I used to sit behind on the bus. You know, the guy that would turn around on a packed bus and call me names at the top of his voice and then laugh really loud.

Maybe he'd had a ball off too, maybe he'd had both off, is that what it does to you? Would I go mad? Was I going mad? Is this a dream, mind you what kind of a person dreams of having a testicle off and masturbating with a bloke with red and yellow clogs on and to boot, getting a lift with the wife and neighbour to the event. My body was aching, aching from doing nothing and my mind was playing tricks. Having time at home feeling unwell was made worse knowing I couldn't go out and do anything, there was only so much day time TV I could stomach. I had lots of time to think of what might happen. Would my partner stay with me if I couldn't give her children? The chemotherapy had wiped me out, if I feel this bad what's it done to my sperm? My mind was now working overtime. If we ever split up, who was going to go out with a bloke with one ball? Again I thought back to my school days, and the bullying that was dished out to someone who was seen as different. Maybe that's why I tried to laugh about it, cover it all up, mention it first, joke about it, so no one would be cruel to me. I had to realise I was a man now and I hadn't been at school for 18 years or so. I started to worry that there was a stigma with having just the one testicle and that I was now a lesser man.

As my confidence grew, the acceptance came soon after, I wasn't really any different from before my operation, apart from a small ball of flesh hanging from my body, my ball had gone.......so what I thought. I still had one and it hit me that I had a choice. I could stay moping about, feeling sorry for myself or I could get on with getting better. I am still me, only I am just a little different.

I realised that having only one testicle was really unimportant, if I had 17 balls it wouldn't really matter. I'm still the same, yes with 17 balls I would struggle to get a pair of Y fronts that fit, but I would still manage. I could go and work in a circus and show off my wad of bollocks. *"Ladies and Gentlemen, the incredible knacker man with 17 TESTICLES, watch how he makes them dance in front of your very eyes."* I could number them all and have the audience pay for a number and pull out a ticket. The first bollock to pop out of my pants with their number on gets to shake the pack.

If I got fed up at the circus, I could paint them dark green and put them in a country show as a sprig of broccoli. The opportunities were there to be explored. What's the worst that could happen I thought? .... coming second to the bloke with 3 parsnips down his trousers on the next table, yes, there is always someone worse off than you.

Chapter 42

GETTING BETTER AND BACK TO HOSPITAL

As my strength slowly returned, so did my appetite. At this point I began to feel better about myself. I was vomiting less and less, and was feeling more optimistic about the future. Negative feelings would pop up now and again but my friends and family made a big difference to how I felt.

Cookridge Hospital the place where I had my chemotherapy was an old red bricked building and although I was to find out just how much love and care there was there, the place still scared me rigid. My first impression was one of fear. One of the nurses had mentioned to my partner that I looked so petrified that my face had drained of all colour – I was ashen. Oh how right he was!. This was the unknown, a place where I'd have to spend a fair bit of time having my treatment, X-rays, having bloods taken and going through the trial. This was a different kind of hospital, a cancer hospital. This was a place full of emotion. At the beginning I was there on a regular basis, having my bloods taken checking to see if it was clear of cancer and having full x-rays and chats with the doctors on how I felt. It was a very solemn place; the one to one care for the patients from the nurses was amazing. I didn't like the place, from the minute I clapped eyes on the old red bricked building. It was fear, fear of the unknown; I had no idea what my future held. My first appointment went in a blur; whatever anyone said to me didn't register. The nurse, that attended to me was being really polite and trying to reassure me that everything was going to be alright. I was trying to listen but my eyes were wandering around the room looking at the other patients and their families. I was to have an appointment with my surgeon who advised me of my situation. He also told me if there was any more cancer in my body. X-rays would follow along with blood tests. This happened on each and every visit. The blood is then sent away and examined to see if there are any cancerous cells in it. I've never been fond of needles but surprisingly you do get used to it, if you think it might save your life, the thought of being afraid of a needle suddenly vanishes. I was surprised by how many people were waiting; all of them had some kind of cancer or were relatives or friends of patients. Some people looked really comfortable sat there; they were probably used to it.

An 11 o'clock appointment usually got called at 12.30pm – 1pm. No one seemed to mind. There seemed to be a feeling of appreciation, people knew that they would be a while so they sat quietly reading papers and magazines. This was a place where people's emotions come out, not just the people with cancer but their family and friends. How could you possibly put a time limit on an appointment like the kind that took place here? People just sat there patiently waiting for their turn and their name to be shouted out.

Although I didn't feel it straight away I soon realised that it was a place of caring, a place where families can be together, where they can listen to advice from the specialists who have their best interests at heart. I looked around the room and there was not one empty seat. It was to be like this every Wednesday. I realised early on that there was an enormous amount of people affected by cancer in this small corner of West Yorkshire. There were obviously lots of these kind of hospitals in the world and it seemed that everyone in that room had a connection; they'd all probably felt fear...

It wasn't a hospital just for testicular cancer; there were all types of cancers in this room. Young ladies, young lads, middle aged mums and dads. Lads in their early 20s, with baseball caps covering bald heads. Everyone had a kind of peace about them, as if they knew there was nothing to complain about, as if they were happy to be alive and appreciating the chance of getting better and getting back to living a normal healthy life.

It was a place where good and bad news coexisted. Patients and families were told how their cancer had responded to treatment. Were they getting better? Or is more treatment required. How can you put a time limit on that? People need time in these situations. A couple in their early 30s, with 2 children aged about 10 and 12 came out of an appointment room, directly in front of me. All four had tears in their eyes. In despair they unite and walk slowly together. I looked to the floor and felt for them. Who ever had the cancer, which ever one of them had been diagnosed; it had the same affect on all four of them. The emotions are raw and unexpected. I had no idea who they were, but I felt for them and often wondered about them. I felt awkward sitting so close to them, as if I was intruding in their time of need.

It seemed to have an effect on the whole room. It was as if it reminded everyone in there, of the time they were told, that they or a loved one had cancer. It was always a blessing when the end of my appointment came. It couldn't come quick enough. It was a caring hospital, but it was a place that reminded me of the reality that cancer had touched my life once again.

Chapter 43

GETTING BETTER WITH THE HELP OF FRIENDS

My neighbour would drive me to the Wednesday appointments. He knew the way there,*" How come you know the way Bill"?* I once asked, *"I came here years ago, with the wife's brother, it ended up beating him."* I went quiet and stared out of the window, another reminder of how many are touched by cancer.

I had a choice, get on with it or mooch about and feel sorry for myself, there could only be one answer to that inner question I posed myself, that afternoon..
I shot myself !

After amazingly surviving the shooting I made a pact with myself that I would donate the weapon to charity and try to remain optimistic, whatever the outcome of my ordeal. I was then sworn in as president of my local gun club.

I've had my ball off; I've had my chemotherapy and survived a shooting, so things were looking up. Every now and then I would get the odd twinge from the shrapnel wedged in my remaining testicle, but other than that life was getting better and certainly worth living for again.

On Christmas Eve one of the lads (Tazmo) decided he'd take me out for a few pints. I'd started drinking quite a bit of the black stuff, Guinness. I felt I needed building up a bit and I'd had my eye on a lovely dress and wanted to be a nice size 8 for the summer! So Guinness had become my tipple. The qualities in Guinness are well documented and the fact it was party time, gave me the perfect excuse to wet my whistle once again with a good friend.

We'd started at lunch time and by mid afternoon we were getting into the spirit of things, when Tazmo came out with a classic. He'd brought up the subject of me only having one testicle. He seemed to take great pleasure from the fact that he had a nice pair of healthy balls and I didn't. It was as if he had opened one of his Christmas presents early and unwrapped one of the oldest joke books known to man. His delivery seemed to tickle him and I enjoyed the fact he was enjoying himself, even though it was at my expense.

As we began to play pool the beer in his body began to affect the jokes that came out of it as he got cruder and louder and he seemed to fill with confidence as I became his victim. Strangely he suddenly had a fascination with pointing his index finger in the direction of my crutch, as he delivered his punch lines. Such classics as *"Set the balls up mate….if there's one missing you'd better tell the landlord"* followed by cackling drunken laughter. Every one potted and I was reminded of another ball lost *"there goes another one, and another and another "*.

175

"I'm starting to sympathise with you and I've just lost 7 balls" as he finally potted the black and won the game. A fit of giggles then took over as he struggled to spit out what he wanted to say next. His laughter was infectious and I was curious to hear what he was struggling to deliver.

There we both were laughing our heads off, him knowing what he was laughing at and me laughing at him laughing at me. Trying to get it out of him was a struggle. He was by now bent over the pool table holding his sides with tears rolling down his face. The other people in the pub had took notice of the laughing and sat with embarrassed smiles.

Finally it came out *"How funny would it be if you got it again in your good knacker."….* I thought I had heard every one in the book by now but this one took the biscuit.

He laughed as though his life depended on it. He laughed so hard that he looked in pain, he laughed and laughed until he keeled over, holding his sides. I couldn't help but laugh back at him; I think I was in shock at his sick sense of humour. But how could I possibly be offended? Whether he knew it or not, he was in the middle of paying me an enormous compliment. He was being himself and had shown me that he felt comfortable in my presence laughing at my plight. He was showing me that he knew I had to keep laughing and he was reminding me that I had indeed set the tone, that somehow, somewhere along the way I had acted in the same way to deal with what I was going through. If I was prepared to laugh at the situation I found myself in, then the people that know and care about me have exactly the same right. If it helped me, then surely it would help them. I'm no hero, far from it, but if there was one thing I could call upon for help when in a difficult or embarrassing situation, it would be laughter. Good old British humour. It helped in the school yard with bullies all those years ago and it backed me up again, when I found that losing part of my anatomy made me feel a lesser man.

I simply had to keep laughing. Trying to have fun, whatever name you wish to put on it. Somewhere on my journey along the way I had read the words *"laughter feeds the soul"*....My old pal Cock knew this all those years ago and I had learned from him. There was no way my soul was going to go hungry. This had to be my mantra, the words I had to try and live by.

I had been doing this for most of my life anyway, usually without much thought. I wore humour like a mask, covering up insecurities. I could have been offended, but how could I be, he was having too much fun for me to stop him. I was laughing at my mate laughing at the thought that if I got it again I would have no balls at all. He found this highly amusing. I shook my head and laughed back at him as he was quite clearly having a right good giggle at my expense. We both agreed he was sick, but if there is one thing that the British are good at its having a good giggle at themselves. *"What did you say to him?"* the landlord asked. *"I'll let him explain when he's calmed down."* We laughed all afternoon and into the night.

It's comforting that I have such warm caring friends! Being able to look on the bright side and joke about a serious issue has allowed my circle of friends to discuss the issues connected to testicular cancer and it's created an awareness of the disease. I know of one such close friend who overcame their fears and visited the doctor when discovering a lump in one of their testicles. Thankfully everything was ok and **she** was given the all clear, *she's a lovely girl, I must catch up with her when I have finished writing this book, I often wonder how she's doing....* Yes it's sick; what my mate Tazmo came out with, but it left a good memory of a great day. *"Merry Christmas for 1999....you arsehole "*

This is the same friend who brought out much needed tears in my adult life. A couple of weeks into my diagnosis I was sitting on my bed at home and the tears began to flow. His partner, another good friend of mine, who likes a good giggle, had been on the phone to my girl to see how I was getting on. In the conversation she'd brought it up how upset he was that his friend had been diagnosed with cancer. It hadn't dawned on me that my friends may be upset. I walked slowly to the bedroom and staring into one of the two mirrors on the wall in front started to cry. It suddenly hit me,*" the hurt it hit like a dog down a pit" and when it comes; it comes, like a steam train*. I was moved that a grown man, a friend of mine was concerned for me. This was the straw that broke the camel's back. Do my friends really think that much of me? Men don't seem to communicate in that way. I was overwhelmed and the tears began to flow. My partner came and sat with me, my head now on her lap. *"Darling what's the matter"?* Through the tears I explained that I was deeply touched that a mate of mine had been upset when hearing about my diagnosis.

To this day I think about this moment. For again without knowing it, he unwittingly did me an enormous service through his caring. He unleashed months of pent up hidden emotion. Feelings that really do need to find a way out. I cried, it wasn't for long, but it was enough to release the tension that had built up. I cried for my mum, for my partner and for the shock of realising just how much people care. I cried for the times I couldn't cry and for the anger that I thought I could hide. Again it brought it home to me just how this illness touches many people.

Chapter 44

BACK ON THE BOOZE

Not long after the diagnosis I was in town with the lads. Everyone was trying to be as normal as possible; I on the other hand thought everyone was looking at me. It was something my mother had also touched on after her diagnosis; she had gone around the local supermarket in a bit of a daze, doing the family shopping. How does that sound? Seven years before when she herself was told she had cancer...she went supermarket shopping for the family, on her return from the hospital. It sounds like madness, but her attitude was that she had to carry on. Tough as old boots she was and still is. We couldn't hold her down if we tried. Don't get me wrong I would have gone with her, but she would insist that she was fine and quite capable. *"I'm not an invalid you know"* she'd say.

Cancer brings out the fighter in you. Up and down each isle she went trying to do what she used to do week in, week out. She'd said the same, she was trying to be normal, but she felt everyone knew she had cancer and everyone was looking at her. In her own words *"she felt as though she had fleas"* It's not only a physical disease, it also affects you mentally.

We shared a few of the same emotions in our own private battles. The lads were at the bar, it was a Thursday night and the town centre boozer was buzzing. The lads were laughing, some showing off, a few of the nutters dancing and everyone was happy. I was fine just looking round the room, then it hit me again, I was stood on my own amongst strangers and I felt like I didn't belong. Mums words began to haunt me. Had I got fleas? I didn't want to be there in the slightest, it wasn't the drink, as I knew full well that booze can alter your mood. I've had a few over the years and knew when it put me on a downer, I found myself staring above the crowded pub. I was not smiling and when I don't smile I'm an ugly bastard. There's nothing pretty about a bloke with a face the shape of an axe, especially when he's frowning or looking sad.

I was well and truly in a world of my own. I looked at the doors, concentrated on the exit signs, then glanced at the lads, who were still oblivious to my feelings and knew that if I said I was going, they wouldn't let me.

They'd always talk you round and give a drunk a good reason to stay. These men were characters and you had to be sharp to play the game.

I was in two minds, then thought bollocks I'm off, I can't do this, everyone laughing, everyone joking. I was mentally exhausted and maybe I should just have been polite and refused to go out in the first place. I finished my beer and looked for somewhere to put my empty glass. Unbeknown to me, Birchy, a real man's man, probably the craziest one out of all of us and the Daddy of the group had his eye on me. *"I'm off Birchy"* It was only early but I'd had enough. *"Come with me, two minutes, that's all I ask"*. I was reluctant to follow him, but I did all the same, as daft as he was, he's a man who demands respect. With his arm on my shoulder he guided me through the busy pub, he didn't speak, but this man knew what he was doing.

Through the drinkers, who stood shoulder to shoulder, and back to back I was led, not knowing where to or why. Eventually we stopped, and I was introduced to a man with a friendly face, he was a tall stocky man's man. *"This is Kean, he's just had his bollock, off....... testicular cancer"* The man held his hand out and I shook it. Not knowing why I had been taken to him in the first place especially as I was adamant I wanted to go home. He left me standing there with a stranger as he made his way back through the crowd to the rest of the lads. He knew what he was doing. For the man he left me with started to talk and asked if I was ok, *"I'm sound mate, but I'm just getting off"* He had a friendly face *"You've just had some unfortunate news about cancer haven't you"?* I nodded but was not in the mood to discuss it with someone who would not understand how I was feeling. For once I was reluctant to talk about it. *"I've had exactly the same as you, about 12 months ago, I had a knacker removed and I'm absolutely sound. I had the works, chemo X-rays the lot and I'm fine."* I was standing next to a man mountain, this bloke was about 6'2" and built like a brick shithouse, he went onto to tell me that he'd indeed had testicular cancer and the treatments that went with it. He reassured me that I would be absolutely fine. The timing of Birchy's gesture was perfect. He'd seen I was struggling, from afar; he'd picked up on the fact that someone was there to help, and then simply left us to get on with it. We chatted for about half an hour, we joked about swapping Y fronts and all the other one liners he'd used and heard. Suddenly I had forgotten that I was feeling low and wanting to go home.

Right there and then I stopped feeling sorry for myself when I realised that life does go on. There in front of me was a bloke who'd gone through exactly the same thing as I was embarking on and he lifted me, when I needed lifting. He didn't even know me. He answered questions that I had not dared to ask anyone and I was flattered that he took the time to help me. We shook hands and I was back on track. Birch did me an enormous favour that night. I've thanked him but like any great man, he felt he didn't really do anything special, but to me he had helped me on my way .With a smile and a shrug of his shoulders he accepted my gratitude. I'm blessed with great friends.

Chapter 45

NEWCASTLE WITH DUCK HEAD

Birchy is the same bloke that had me in stitches in Newcastle.

It was a stag do a couple of years after my diagnosis. I now had a few self inflicted nick names and could be known as one of the following, 1 knack, Adolf or Testi. We were all waiting in the pub, well before 9am in the morning and some of the lads were well into their third pint. The bus was late and the best man was getting some stick from the lads, he went on look out in the car park for the phantom bus. Ten minutes later he popped his head around the pub door "no worries boys; it's arrived, wait until you see the driver." In he walked "Duck Head, the coolest bus driving pensioner in the west. By the end of the trip he would be pushing 70, pushing his luck or pushing his bus. Proudly he sported a whiter than white ducks arse hair cut, the tip of his quiff touched the tip of his chin. Oh did I feel sorry for this bloke, I knew he was going to get some stick. But did he care...not a bit. The word cool had been written for this man. He was draped in a classic Reg Varney style uniform .The pale blue 1950's style bus driver's jacket and big badge to match on his lapel gave him his own identity. He was born to drive.... His look was complete with one pair of navy blue slacks with a crease sharp enough to cut glass and a pair of black plastic shoes adorned with a centre metre French flag on either side. His look was as sharp as his tongue. When he walked into the pub; the whole lot of us cracked up. He was immediately christened "Duck Head", within minutes 40 blokes quack quacked at the top of their voices. We were in hysterics. He gave us a look that said he didn't care less. Oh how these people earn their money.

One of the lads came running in from the car park *"You should see the state of his bus, it's older than Duck Head"* with that another rousing laugh and a chorus of *"quack, quack". "Come on Duck Head are we off pal",* cried one of the lads *"I'm not going anywhere until I've had a pint,"* came his reply. He was an instant hit. He'd done this job a thousand times and was ready for whatever came at him.

The bus was an amazing experience, straight out of a 1950,s movie, pale blue to match his jacket and enough room on the dashboard to rest his quiff while he drove. We knew from the off that this would be a good trip. Every time Duck Head reversed his back door would come open and an alarm would start bleeping, every time it bleeped 40 screaming quack quack chants came back at him. He took it like a duck and gave as good as he got. As soon as we set off, a shout from the back of the bus to set fire to the driver was heard, he didn't bat an eyelid. He's seen and heard it all before.

On the motorway and half an hour into the trip Duck head very kindly allowed the lads to line up at the side of his bus to empty their bladders. Whilst we were parked up Duck Head got stuck into the booze, this guy didn't' care. He was on about his 3rd bottle of WKD, a blue Alco pop, when one of the quieter members of our group, questioned him. *"Do you think it's a good idea mate, drinking that booze while you're driving",* Duck head flicked his quiff in his direction" *Why, what do you mean?" "Well what about your license"?* He took another long mouthful from his bottle, paused and replied *"What f****** licence"?* The bus erupted. He was the star of the show. We'd just got settled and off again when I shouted out from the back of the bus " *I can't believe there's 79 testicles on this bus",* , feeling quite pleased with myself at a very poor joke, when Birchy replied, *"why, have you got 3?"* Everyone was laughing; the banter was now flying around the bus *"Stop at a pond Duck Head, if you need a paddle".* His beak remained tightly shut. It was a crazy weekend and we all took the driver to our hearts.

We even had a collection for him and presented him with a loaf of bread. He saw the funny side. He did get the last laugh though. Two or three weeks after the trip, the best man who'd arranged everything got a nasty little surprise on his visa card. Duck Head had a lavish evening meal at the hotel a full English breakfast and a rather large bar bill put on the best man's visa. These were the times that helped to pull me through, to laugh and to make me realise that friends and acquaintances can really lift your spirits. At the end of the trip I was the last off the bus. I'd watched everyone shake Duck Heads wing as they thanked him for the great trip. When it was my turn to leave the bus, I reached out my hand to shake his webbed fingers." *By the way, what is your real name"* I enquired"? He came close and whispered in my ear......... ***"Donald** and if you tell your mates, you won't have any bollocks left to scratch".* With that he winked and lit a cigarette. I shook his wing and laughed as I walked across the car park. I had met my very own Donald Duck. It was so important for me to have friends around me and thankfully for me they have all joined in the banter about me losing a testicle. Some have even commented that it has helped them and stopped them feeling awkward in my company. I know it's not everyone's cup of tea to joke about what they have been through, but humour is a wonderful tonic and is a universal language. I should know when you have a face as funny looking as mine, people laugh at you whatever language they speak.

Chapter 46

DENIAL

When I was diagnosed with testicular cancer I was in denial. It couldn't possibly happen to me. I was a young man with a lot of life to look forward to. I didn't accept it, I didn't want to. I dealt with it by blanking it out and trying to laugh about the situation. I can't speak for everyone that has been touched by the illness., It wouldn't be right to, but from talking to people who have a connection with it I have found that once they have adjusted at their own pace to the reality of the situation, they then find an amazing strength to fight this condition.

The denial my own mother showed came in the form of being diagnosed and being too busy to have cancer. She admitted that she was in denial when she was first given the results that she was indeed suffering from cancer and she would need treatment. She at first confirmed to herself that it was a mistake. She believed they were talking to someone else, as it didn't register with her. She didn't want to hear it, she didn't cry and she thought they'd made a terrible mistake, why would they diagnose her with breast cancer when she felt perfectly well. The doctor *said "you can cry if you want", * mum replied*" but why,".* She then looked at the female nurse and asked, "*does he mean me?, Does he mean I've got cancer?" "Yes"* came the reply, she didn't wish to hear "*Oh, I can't have, I've got my holiday to Corfu booked and I've got to go to Argos to pick up a hat and coat stand as we're moving house".*

They then took her, still in a state of denial and confusion to another room, where they tried to convince her and comfort her in the best way possible, with honesty and compassion.

That night when she got us all together to break the news, she tried to convince us that it was a mistake; it was as if she was trying to protect herself and her family. The next morning she woke up with tears slowly rolling down her cheek. In her own words, she still didn't believe it. When she had to get back to hospital on the day of her results, she was told by the nurse that her friends were also there, waiting for their own results. Mum was confused. *"What friends?"* These were the ladies she had met the day she had tests for cancer. They had gone through the same tests at the same time and laughing and joking on the day. Three out of four were to be diagnosed with breast cancer. *"Well we did laugh"* said mum, *"I think we were all in denial, but the humour helped us".*

Chapter 47

EVEN MORE HOPE

These are mums words ... A smoking room in a Hospital pre smoking ban !! *"The four of us, all strangers, went to sit in the smoking room at the hospital and had a right good chin wag; it was as if we were waiting for a bus. We had all just been given our results of our tests and we were all sharing the same experience. The first lady spoke, what's up with you,? as she took a cigarette out of her handbag and put it to her lips. Breast cancer, (1) we all looked sullen, what's up with you? came the question firing the same one back, puffing the smoke into the room and looking up to the ceiling, breast cancer, she says (2) I lit a cigarette and took a puff, the same lady asked me what was up with me, breast cancer, (3) again we all looked sullen, the mood was sombre. I then asked the same question to the lady who hadn't spoken yet, what's up with you love? Her eyes looked at all of us one by one, as she spoke, PILES, and the whole room erupted into fits of laughter".*

Mum says the next hour flew in that room as she said she hadn't laughed like that for ages. The human spirit was working over that day. The lady with piles apologised that it wasn't as serious and went onto say she felt awful that she only had piles and again laughter filled the room. These ladies had their own therapy.

Chapter 48

SPIRIT

A friend of mine whose own mother is currently going through her own battle with cancer told a similar tale of his mum's humour, helping not only her but the people around her. He has since left his job to care for her.

"Mum was in hospital wired up to a machine and we'd had a call to say that she was not at her best. I am an only child and very close to her, myself and my father thought we had been called to the hospital to say our last goodbyes as she had been fighting it for some time.

Dad and I were emotional and the strain of thinking that we might not be seeing her again tore us apart. But as we sat around the bed in silence my eyes fixed on dad's as we both feared the worst. She was wired up to a machine and didn't look well......she then breaks the silence "I feel like that bloody game", "game" we said? Unsure of what she meant, Yeah, you know that with all the things sticking out of it. KER PLUNK, we all laughed." He told me the story and I could feel the passion for his mum's plight in his every word. *"Here she is my mum, my invincible mum, the lady I thought would be here for ever, and sat wired up to some machine and she can still come out with a great one liner."*

His eyes were filling up. It was another tale of humour acting as a tonic, not only for the patient, but the person's immediate family.

Chapter 49

THE GOOD NEWS

I am writing this to let everyone know that there is life after cancer, the good news is that testicular cancer is almost always curable if found early. The disease responds well to treatment even if it has spread to other parts of the body. These days more than 9 out of 10 patients are cured, most of them enjoy a normal sex life, that includes myself, if you can call me normal, as I'm quite partial to dressing up as a scuba diver and chasing the other half around the house, throwing crab sticks in her direction , purely for my own enjoyment of course. If you wish to participate in this pass time, always consult the wife, get her to wear protective clothing, a heavy duty welder's mask or 1923 cast iron diving helmet is usually a good option as this cuts down on any potential eye injuries.

The downside to this sexual activity is that by the time you've got your suit off the urge to perform has usually gone. Secondly an erection in a wet suite is quite restricting. You could however slit the rubber to allow for penetration, but please don't wear it to go surfing in

Cornwall as you may receive some strange looks from other beach goers.

Please don't get the wrong impression that any treatment I have received to cure my condition has had an effect on my mental health. Apart from having a testicle missing I would call myself quite normal. Despite the fact that at the moment there is a lawsuit going on with the Cat's solicitors who are trying to prove I have been abusing him with a mallet, and of course I totally deny all allegations. It is also untrue that I forced him to sit at my desk whilst I wrote, using his rear end as a pencil sharpener and pen holder. I deny every aspect of every comment put to me; I am both hurt and angry at these lies aimed in my direction. As I write this, the cat is sat in his basket flicking through its solicitor's notes. I know he wants me out of here so he can rule the roost, I know he would love to reclaim his place in the master bedroom, snuggled up to my girl. He thinks I haven't noticed the way he licks its rear end and gives me one of those leering glances late on in the evening, just before I throw it out. Let's be straight, about one thing I'm not a weirdo, slightly different I may be, but everyone is entitled to be their own person. What works for one might not work for another. But I do know I had some pretty crazy thoughts. Was I going to die? Cancer or the word cancer does that to you. I felt overwhelmed that I had been told I had cancer; it was probably made harder as it only seemed like yesterday that I'd heard my mother getting the same news. At the time it didn't seem to matter that the cure rate for testicular cancer was very high if it was found early, as it usually is with this kind of cancer.

Many emotions arise, emotions I thought I had long lost; confusion can set in along with frequent changes of mood. This no doubt puts a strain on other aspects of your life. I didn't experience feelings in a particular order and I am sure the next man wouldn't go through exactly the same thought process as me, but all the same the same feelings may occur. There is no right way to feel, no wrong way to feel. People's reactions differ. Family and friends sometimes need as much support as the diagnosed person. The same fears crop up, will I lose a loved one? I'd rather it be me. There is guidance and support out there if you choose to take it, it's a wise decision but again it's up to the individual.

Chapter 50

ORDINARY PEOPLE

On one of my many visits to have yet another chest x-ray, I was sat in the waiting room with my clothes in a basket draped in a hospital robe, sipping an irresistible drink for 45 minutes, around 4 pints of the stuff. This shows up as a dye in your x-ray and shows if you're clear from cancer. You sit supping it until it's all gone and then you're in for your x-ray and examination. Two hours can be along time, but especially with a pair of legs like mine hanging out of the bottom of the dressing gown.

The man sat next to me was about 20 years older than me and he was in the early stages of his diagnosis. The poor man was a blithering wreck. Now I know I can talk and go on a bit, but I think it must have been the fear and panic in him that had taken over. He never stopped talking about how frightened he was. He was talking uncontrollably about how his wife and children might cope should he die, the fact he's only 55 and he'd got so many plans for the rest of his life. The fact he'd kept himself fit, he walked a lot, that there was no history in his family of cancer and that he was unsure what the hospital was going to do to him. I genuinely felt for this man, I tried to reassure him that he would be ok, I didn't know, but I'd explained I'd lost a testicle within the last year and that the tests are still clear and that I've been fine. He was in the early stages and quite clearly frightened. I wanted to help him, I tried to reassure him, but his questions were coming at me too fast, by the time I'd started to answer one question, he'd hit me with another. I thought the best way was to just let him get on with it. He wouldn't allow me to reassure him. It helped him by just letting it out, whether he wanted to hear me speak or not.

He was wearing his heart on his sleeve that day and the fear was coming through thick and fast. His eyes darted around the room towards anyone that he thought might listen, some tried to reassure him, some gave a half smile and some kept flicking through magazines. *"You just never know do you"*, he went on. How he could even think about getting any serious conversation out of me, with the way I must have looked, baffled me. Self conscious doesn't come into it. I'm draped in a white dressing gown, sipping the purple stuff with my supermarket basket at my feet, adorned with all my day's possessions and two bits of string for legs hanging down from the dressing gown.

I've always thought about this man and wondered how he was doing. Seeing my legs, dangling down as if hanging out of a birds nest may have added to his anxiety, I could empathise with this stranger and I'm sure the other people in the waiting room felt the same. I felt for him. We'd all been there; at some point or other and all dealt with it in our own way. Some people bottle it up, some never stop talking, some laugh about and some surround themselves with people who understand, there's not one certain way of coping, but everyone empathised with him, no one felt he was embarrassing himself, we are all human beings, we all feel fear.

My own emotions were still a bit erratic, once the realisation came knocking in my mind, many feelings would surface. How, it's great to be alive, back down to I'm a eunuch with one knacker and a lesser man. My checks at the hospital were coming back clear and I was getting on with life. I would soon be going back to work and getting back to normal. The first few weeks I was allowed to go back part time to break myself in gently. I was very grateful for this and felt I was ready for some normality.

On my first morning I had got half way to work, approached a roundabout, when I should have taken a left turn but I just kept driving round and around the roundabout. I went round one more time and then pulled up in a lay by. I realised I was not yet ready to face the questions of my colleagues, and just at that moment the whole cancer thing hit me between the eyes. I sat in my car just looking ahead. After about 20 minutes I drove home and as I walked through the door, I told my partner *"I just can't do it, I'm not ready"*. She said I looked grey and rang work for me.

I thought I was capable, I felt fit but the emotional side of the illness had reared its ugly head again. I felt a failure and was back in limbo; work was fine about me not going in so I arranged to go in the following week. Eventually I went back part time and gradually building my hours up each week. Everyone was great at work although I did feel awkward when questions of where I had been and how come I'd been off work for three months were put to me by colleagues. At that time I was too emotionally raw to discuss losing a testicle to cancer so I said that I'd had problems in my groin. I was getting used to the half days and slowly slotting in but felt a bit guilty to the full time staff, which were getting most of the work to do in my absence. You can't put a time limit on how someone can come round after cancer, both physically and emotionally, I felt anger along with guilt that I'd been letting people down.

I did gradually work my way up to full time work again and would often daydream of setting fire to the manager's desk for allowing me to come back to a busy office. I even considered arranging a strip-o-gram wrestler for her as a reward for her caring nature. I'd stare out of the window with visions of this 23 stone hairy brute sticking his thumb in her ear whilst he pushed her head against her desk. He'd bounce on her in full view of the office; he'd be screaming submit and have her in a half nelson while people just stepped over her. As he lifted her up in a head lock and drops her to the floor, staff would randomly bounce on her as they passed. I'd then be brought back to earth again as she'd be stood over me demanding to know why I hadn't answered the phone that had been ringing for five minutes.

Time quickly passed and I'd got into the swing of full time work again. I'd still have my mood swings and have thoughts of pity me, followed by how lucky I was. I'd laugh with the lads about my knacker and within 3 months of my operation, started to get back into my football. Whether it was the extra zest for life that spurred me on I will never know but I had this almighty urge for not wanting to miss out on anything. As if I had been give a second chance. I'd started training with the team again and the lads were amazed that I was back so soon. I started as a substitute and was told in front of the lads by the manager that *"You'll go on the right wing, as close to the touchline as you can, because you've lost your left testicle, your balance won't be as good and now all your weight is on your right side, I don't want you drifting across the pitch when you run with the ball".*

Everyone laughed out loud. True to his word, and I thought he was joking; he put me on the right wing. When I walked on to the pitch I felt on top of the world, I was knackered, the chemo does wipe you out, but I was elated. I was back doing something I loved. I was nicknamed womble in the changing room and all the usual one liners were flying about. I blamed a few missed chances on my balance, due to my missing testicle but now my life was going forward.

In the pub after the game a few of the lads were curious and wanted to know how I'd found I had testicular cancer. I was straight with them and said if I hadn't had gone to the doctor, who knows what might have happened. There was and still is a stigma with men both young and old on checking themselves out. By the seriousness of their faces I knew there was concern that it could happen to anyone. With a bit of luck, the very fact I had started living my life again, playing football, socialising having fun and talking about my experience has had a positive effect on this delicate illness. My pal's have laughed, some have cried and we have discussed openly the condition and it's all awareness. This has to be good.

As time passed I'd be summoned to hospital every 6 months, have my blood taken, have a chat with my surgeon and he'd ask about my well being, my family, partner and how I felt. It was again good to talk, he'd also examine me and the old smell of the rubber gloves would invade the air and remind me of the first bloke who'd originally scanned my ball. I'd get a thorough examination, my groin; my one and only ball, my back, my neck and my chest would be x-rayed. This would always be followed by having my bloods taken, to see if there was any cancer in the body. On my visits I became less and less frightened and became more appreciative of my good fortune. I'd sit in the room and again it would be about an hour to an hour and a half behind schedule, but no one minded. I'd look at the other people in the room, the guys with the bald heads and their baseball caps. I'd look at the parents, the wives and partners of the patients and I'd see their worry and concern etched on their faces. How they'd grip their loved ones arms and sense a different kind of love. I'd look and think back to when I was in their shoes, frightened of being so afraid. Afraid of the future and what was going to happen. Don't get me wrong I was still pretty frightened, frightened that the cancer could come back. But as time went on I was getting more comfortable with having had cancer.

There was always the fear that if I've had it once I could get it again, but I'd vowed not to dwell on thoughts of this kind. After each appointment and the checks on my bloods, I'd go home and get on with life and wait for the results. In a couple of days I'd get a brown envelope with my next 6 monthly appointments. This meant I was fine. It was always on my mind, how I'd coped if it came back negative, but I'd resolved to dealing with that, if and when it happened.

Acceptance of a situation can be mistaken for bravery, who wants to be known as brave when you would rather not be in that situation at all....maybe that explains it better. For the people that I have known who have been touched by this disease have hinted that people have called them brave and felt awkward and denied they were. But it's not about being brave, it's far from it, it's about acceptance, accepting that you have had or have still got cancer and getting on with it.

On a couple of occasions after my latest visit, the alarm bells were ringing when I'd either get a phone call from the hospital or a note asking if I could attend the next Wednesday clinic as my bloods had come back abnormal. This always concerned me and the same feelings would surface, the same ones that were there when I was originally diagnosed. I'd try not to dwell on it, but it was always there at the back of my mind. If I'd had any medication or been on the beer or had a bout of flu before my routine visit, as it could affect my results and my blood could show up abnormal.

The nurses were always wonderful when they rang to tell me about the findings and always reassured me that they were there if required. It is a comfort to know that whatever they find, they react to it straight away. They always give you an honest explanation and you genuinely feel their compassion for their career and patients. You stay in remission for the first 10 years after your initial diagnosis. I had bi annual appointments that eventually would go to annual. On the tenth year, you're finally given the all clear and this happened in 2009 ironically it was the day of my birthday.

As time went on I started to think about my frozen sperm in the hospital and whether or not I could father a child. I'd try not to worry too much about it and just let life lead me to wherever I was meant to go. I'd see people with their children and temporarily feel sorry for myself and would wonder if the girlfriend had the same feelings. I'd then try to snap out of it and be grateful for my health.

Chapter 51

MIRACLES DO HAPPEN

I was diagnosed with cancer in December 1998 and in May 2000 I got a phone call at work from my partner. She was in bits on the phone, I was embarrassed in the office as I was trying to console her as I whispered down the phone to try and calm down. Even the wrestler had picked up on it; he'd temporally loosened his grip on the boss's neck and tried to listen into our conversation. She was weeping inconsolably and I was struggling to reassure her. *"Talk slowly I don't understand what you're saying."* I feared the worst, someone must have died. She's had an accident? The cat's shot itself, it had recently joined a gun club and was building up an arsenal in the cellar, it was acting very strange and would go out at all hours wearing a bandana and draped in a gun belt.

"You're going to be so cross, I'm so sorry, I've ruined our lives" All sorts shot through my mind and no it wasn't the cat! What could she have done to ruin our lives? She was inconsolable, had she slept with the vicar again or burned the house down? I had no idea what she'd done,

that could be so awful, and I began to dread the words that were to follow. *"I'm so sorry"*. I was still whispering down the phone, the wrestler had now gone on his break and left the boss tied up by a phone cable suspended from the ceiling,. I knew he'd be back in a while to let her down. I whispered with urgency "sorry for what????"

"I'M   P R E G N A N T"

I paused ...*"are you sure it's yours"*? I could hear the wrestler crying in the back office. He'd been monitoring the call, checking my customer service skills. I repeated the word as if spelling it back. *"You're PREGNANT?"* , She kept repeating the same word ...sorry *"I've ruined our lives"*. A test at the Doctors had confirmed her suspicions'. Yes she was pregnant! I put the phone down after trying to reassure her and the nosey sod in the back office that we would be ok. I was trying to convince all three of us, it was surreal and we agreed to talk when I got home.

As it slowly sunk in I began to feel like a real man.

I gave the wrestler a lift home and decided to drive home naked with the sun roof open. He stroked my face with a feather as we listened to Sweet Caroline on the car stereo. He cried, I cried, there was a pause in the song and Neil Diamond cried. We swayed side to side without speaking and he looked lovingly into my eyes and fanned my beautiful perfect testicle with his cowboy hat. Love on the Rocks came on and we pulled into a lay-by, we sat staring with large grins at my testicle. We were both so proud of him and he really was a beauty. I was soon home and smiling at the neighbours as I locked my car door without a stitch on. I walked through the door, I didn't even open it - we had it repaired a few days later. She stood there, looking at my naked body and the damaged door. She was all bleary eyed and looked so sorry. I walked over and hugged her; we'd been through so much already and now this. I kept asking her if she was really pregnant and we just sat and held each other.

Through her tears she asked who the tit with the cowboy hat was and why was he stroking my testicle.

Our tears mingled and danced down both our cheeks as we held each other, the wrestler now drenched had put his umbrella up.

We'd only ever talked about having a family in passing and still had all the wrigglers tucked up safely if we ever needed them. Thankfully this happened without really trying and as it sunk in, I realised I'd subconsciously been going through some of my own demons. I'd always worried I might not be able to father a child due to the chemotherapy and only having one testicle. The light had begun to reappear in our lives and over the coming days, we both reassured each other that everything would be fine. As the days and weeks passed, the joys of becoming a dad entered my life. We'd both been through a lot and I started to realise just how wonderful this news was.

In January 2001 our joy was complete as my son entered the world, at a wapping 8 pound 5 oz, not bad for a skinny bloke with one ball.

I was at the birth and wept as I realised I had a baby son. We named him Kaius, a wonderful roman name that means "to rejoice"; say no more...he is our miracle. It's wonderful being a father and equally as nice having a pair of balls back in the house!

On March 14th 2009 on my 43rd birthday and 10 years after my diagnosis I was finally discharged and given the green light to go and have a normal life............NORMAL LIFE.......Me !!!

AND FINALLY...
A LITTLE BIT MORE

The wrestler is my son's God father and now lives with my old manager, the cat is in rehab with gunshot wounds, I'm fine, mum's fine, I miss my ball and my old pal cock….Oh and I nearly forgot…...,I'm saving up for a garage to shit behind, just in case my plumbing fails.

The End…………..but wait….there's a bit more……………

THE FACTS

Testicular cancer accounts for approximately 0.7% of all cancers. It's the most common cancer in men between the age of 20 and 35. Approximately 1,960 men are diagnosed with the condition each year in the UK. Around 70 people die every year from testicular cancer.

The testicles are part of the male reproductive system. They produce sperm and the male hormone testosterone. The testicles hang down behind the penis, and are located within the scrotum (a loose bag of skin).

The body is made up of millions of different types of cells. Sometimes these cells can become abnormal and start to multiply. When this happens it causes a growth, known as a tumour, to form. Tumours can be benign (not cancerous) or malignant (cancerous). They can occur in any part of the body where the cells multiply abnormally.

Testicular cancer is different from many other types of cancer. Most cancers tend to affect older people. Testicular cancer, however, is more common in young and middle-aged men. Approximately 50% of all cases of testicular cancer affect men who are under 35 years of age, and 90% of cases affect those who are under the age of 55.

Cancer of the testicles is also one of the most treatable forms of cancer. Over 95% of men make a full recovery from testicular cancer.

Kean Turner

ALERT ALERT ALERT ALERT ALERT ALERT ALERT ALERT ALERT ALERT ALERT ALERT ALERT ALERT ALERT ALERT ALERT ALERT

Warning signs

The early signs of testicular cancer are usually obvious and easy to spot, watch out for one or more of these:

- A hard lump on the front or side of your testicle.
- Swelling or enlargement of testicle.
- Pain or discomfort in a testicle or in the scrotum (this is the sack that holds the testicle). I've met a few of these in my time!
- An unusual size difference between one testicle and the other.

Other warning signs may include:

- A heavy feeling in the scrotum
- A dull ache in the lower stomach, groin or scrotum. This is the one that prompted my good self to pop to the doctors.

TYPES OF TESTICULAR CANCER

There are two main types of testicular cancer:
Seminoma, and non-Seminoma

The terms Seminoma and non-Seminoma refer to the type of cell that makes up the cancerous tumour. Seminoma testicular cancers only contain Seminoma cells. Non-Seminomas may contain a variety of different cancer cells. However, both types of testicular cancer are treated in a similar way.

Testicular cancer is also a type of germ cell cancer. A germ cell cancer is one that starts in the cells that are used to make sperm or eggs (ovarian cancer is another type of germ cell cancer).

Treating Testicular Cancer

Testicular cancer is one of the most treatable cancers, with approximately 95% of men making a full recovery. As with most cancers, the earlier the condition is detected and diagnosed, the better your chance of recovery. The three main forms of treatment for testicular cancer are:

- Surgery
- chemotherapy
- radiotherapy.

Surgery is the most common and effective form of treatment for testicular cancer. It is normally the first line of treatment for all stages and types of testicular cancer. Surgery and other treatments for testicular cancer are outlined below.

Chemotherapy

Chemotherapy is a type of cancer treatment that uses anti-cancer medicines to either kill the malignant (cancerous) cells in your body, or stop them multiplying. If your testicular cancer is advanced, or has spread to other places in your body, you may require chemotherapy. It is also used to help prevent the cancer from returning. Chemotherapy is most commonly used to treat non-Seminoma tumours. Chemotherapy medicines can either be injected or given to you orally (by mouth). Chemotherapy can also attack the normal, healthy cells in your body, which is why this form of treatment can potentially have many side effects. The most common side effects include:

- vomiting
- hair loss
- nausea
- mouth sores
- fatigue
-

These side effects are usually only temporary and you should find that they do improve once you have completed your treatment.

Radiotherapy

Radiotherapy is a form of cancer therapy which uses high energy beams of radiation to help destroy cancer cells. Most Seminoma types of testicular cancer will require radiotherapy as well as surgery. This is to help prevent the cancer from returning. If your testicular cancer has spread to your lymph nodes, you may also require radiotherapy. Side effects of this type of treatment can include:

- fatigue
- skin rashes
- stiff joints and muscles
- loss of appetite
- nausea
-

These side effects are usually only temporary, and you should find that they improve once you have completed your treatment.

My Own Treatment Experience - Chemotherapy – Peripheral Meuropathy

Tingling in your hands and feet could result in having difficulty doing up your buttons. Hands and feet could be more sensitive to the cold. Rather like the time I'd been substitute for 90 minutes. I eventually went on, got in position then the ref blew for the end of the game, charming. I couldn't get my shirt buttons fastened in the changing room, so the week after I started to wear tank tops. I searched charity shops for easy to wear garments that matched the football kit. Alternatively you can add a bit of fun to the proceedings by asking your team mates to bring clothes in and then spend your time parading around the pitch looking like a pantomime dame instead of sucking oranges waiting for your chance. Take my advice; gas masks impede your communicating skills when shouting for a pass. I could often be seen leaving the changing room in white wellington boots, PVC yellow hot pants and a blonde wig. A full suit of medieval armour is great for protection and although it did result in me throwing away my 28 year old shin pads it didn't do anything for my pace.

Kidney Infection

Chemotherapy can change the function of your kidneys and I had regular blood tests to see how well my kidneys were working. My kidneys were apparently working well, but occasionally they would ring in sick or change their shifts. It used to drive me mad when they took 2 week holidays and stopped working altogether. Although chemotherapy side effects may be hard to deal with at the time, these side effects will gradually disappear once treatment is over.

Chemotherapy affects people in different ways. Some people find they are able to lead a fairly normal life during their treatment, but many find they become very tired and have to take things much more slowly. With me I think I have always been a little touched in the head and so was born with the side effects. Try not to overdo it though and just do a little to start with and take time to care for yourself. I would advise against 13 cans of Guinness, 2 packets of pork scratchings, 3 quail eggs, 2 tins of peach halves and a brandy snap coated in marmite. Don't blame the chemotherapy for making you vomit if you have this little lot straight after your treatment .

Chest X-Rays

Usually a chest x-ray is done to check for any signs that the cancer has spread to the lungs or to the lymph glands in the abdomen. The CT scan takes a series of x-rays which build up a 3 dimensional picture of the inside of the body. You may be given a drink or injection of a dye which allows particular areas to be seen more clearly.

This was the aniseed drink I had to sip before my x-ray, not very pleasant but obviously worthwhile. I was given an hour to an hour and a half before my x-ray to drink it, this gives enough time for it to work around your body. The only side effect here is maybe feeling a little hot all over for a few minutes, you may also be given an injection instead of the drink. If you are allergic to iodine or have asthma you could have a more serious reaction to the injection, so it's important to let your doctor know beforehand. The scan takes about 10-30 minutes and you're usually allowed home as soon as it's over.

Magnetic Resonance Imaging (MR or NMR Scan)

This test uses magnetism to build up cross-sectional pictures of the body. Some people are given an injection of dye into a vein, sounds a bit barbaric, I know, but these guys really know what they are doing and research is on going all the time against finding a cure or reducing symptoms in cancer patients. The injection can improve the image, giving a clearer picture.

During the test you're asked to lie very still, very difficult for yours truly, hyperactive Ronnie fought the E numbers in my body from far too many blue smarties as a kid. I don't recommend a dose of red bull before this kind of treatment. You're asked to lie very still on a couch inside a long chamber for up to an hour. This can be unpleasant if you don't like enclosed spaces. I felt a bit like Buck Rogers laying there, it's very futuristic; Spock serves you drinks straight after and allows you to rub his ears to calm you down. He also agrees to sign any "Star Trek" memorabilia you may have. There was also a martian playing a mouthorgan who did a great rendition of fly me to the moon, while two dalek's smooched in the corner, When it was all over we all enjoyed a game of twister until one of the darlics struggled to reach the green circle and had to be helped up with a car jack from a passing motorist.

If you get claustrophobic, it may help to mention this to the radiographer. The MRI scanning process is also very noisy but you will be given ear plugs or headphones to wear. It reminded me of Mr and Mrs, the early 80s game show where the wife or hubby had to go in a booth with headsets on and answer questions correctly on their relationship, I didn't do bad. I left my appointment with a set of tea towels, a pan set and 2 tickets for Stars on Ice in Romford. You may even be given the option of taking a tape or CD in with you to make you feel more comfortable. When I turned up with my Cello and 30 piece orchestra the nurse seemed a little perturbed, but she did her best to accommodate us all.

The chamber is a very powerful magnet, so before entering the room you should remove any metal belongings. People who have cardiac monitors' pacemakers or some types of surgical clips cannot have an MRI scan because of the magnetic fields. The nurse made me take off my full suit of armour before I entered the chamber. The pull was that great, an ice cream van entered the room and we all shared a magnum while I played Bach on the cello. The ice cream man got on really well with one of the dalek's and offered him a job; he now does 30 hours a week and works it around his filming schedule. Takings are up, and everything's going well apart from 23 regulars being exterminated in his first two days. Once all tests are carried out, the doctor will have a good idea of the type of cancer and the stage at where it's at (whether it is just within the testicle or spread further).

It will probably take several days for the results of your tests to be ready and a follow up appointment will be made for you. This waiting period can be a very anxious time and it may help to talk things over with a close friend or relative.

Orchidectomy

An Orchidectomy is the medical name for the surgical removal of a testicle. If you have testicular cancer, it is necessary to remove the whole testicle because only removing the tumour may lead to the cancer spreading. Therefore, by removing the entire testicle your chances of making a full recovery are greatly improved. if your testicular cancer is caught in the early stages, an Orchidectomy may be the only treatment that you require. The operation is performed under general anaesthetic. A small cut is made in your groin and the whole testicle is removed through this incision. If you want to, you can have an artificial (prosthetic) testicle inserted into your scrotum, so that the appearance of your testicles is not greatly affected. This artificial testicle is normally made from silicone.

How Will an Orchidectomy Affect Me?

Following an Orchidectomy, you will need to stay in hospital for a few days. If you only have one testicle removed, there should not be any lasting side effects. Your sex life, and your ability to father children, will not be affected. If you have both testicles removed, you will be infertile. However, it is very rare for both testicles to be affected by cancer and, therefore the removal of both is uncommon. You may be able to bank your sperm before your operation, which should allow you to father children if you decide that you want to.

Early Stage Testicular Cancer

In people with early stage testicular cancer, surgery is done with the aim of curing the cancer. Sometimes additional treatment – chemotherapy or radiotherapy is also given to reduce the risks of it coming back. These treatments are successful in curing cancer in over 95% of men.

If The Cancer Does Come Back

It is very rare for testicular cancer to come back, but if that happens, the treatment can again get rid of the cancer in most men.

Advanced Stage

If the cancer comes back again, or has spread widely in the body, further treatment may still be able to get rid of the cancer. There are situations where a cure is not possible, treatment may be able to control the cancer, leading to an improvement in symptoms and a better quality of life. However for some men in this situation the treatment will have no effect upon the cancer and they will get the side effects without any of the benefit. This is the cold side of cancer.

Making decisions about treatment in this situation can be difficult and you may need to discuss in detail with your doctor whether you wish to have treatment. If you choose not to you can still be given supportive (palliative) cure, with medicines to control any symptoms.

Hope - Further treatment for Testicular Cancer

If the cancer has not spread and was completely removed with the testicle, the operation may be the only treatment you will need.

Monitoring

After your operation, it is very important for you to be seen regularly in the outpatient's clinic by your doctor for blood tests, chest x-rays and CT scans. This is because in some patients the cancer may come back in the glands at the back of the abdomen or in the lungs. If your doctor feels that the risk of the cancer returning is very low, you will be seen regularly in the clinic and will not have any further treatment unless your tests show that the cancer has come back. This is known as Surveillance Policy. If the risk of the cancer returning is thought to be higher, further treatment may be given to help prevent it. This is known as Adjuvant Therapy. The type of treatment depends on the type of cancer.

After Treatment

After your treatment has finished, you will have regular check ups, blood tests, scans and x-rays. These will continue for several years. I'm now in my 10th year and have just been discharged along with many, many men. As time passed I started to look forward to my 6 monthly, then yearly examinations, my annual grope. I ached for the smell of rubber gloves and cold alien hands, on my testicle. No not the dalek. Time has passed and in I'm no longer as afraid as I was a few years ago. I've had highs and I've had lows, highs with my friends and seeing my wonderful son born, welcoming a new pair of testicles into the house and lows where my old life as I once knew it would never be quite the same again. My life had changed and I had no control over it. The only control I had was how I would deal with it. I had to have hope. Research shows that people find they can be low and anxious once their treatment has finished.

I remember sitting in our home alone, the cat and my demons for company wondering what it's all about. My mind skipped from being frightened, to elation, thankful that they found the cancer early. It would be just as easy to slip back into feeling sorry for myself. A swift crack of the mallet on the back of the cat's head usually helped to change my train of thought. This cat was wise though as soon as my hand was raised he'd slipped his yellow Gay and Proud crash helmet on before he proceeded to wash both balls.

High Dose Chemotherapy

This involves giving a very high dose of chemotherapy to try and destroy all the testicular cancer cells. This can also damage cells in the bone marrow; certain cells in your blood called peripheral blood stem cells are collected and stored before treatment begins, then returned to the blood afterwards. This is known as stem cell support.

Contraception

It is not advisable to father a child while having any of the chemotherapy drugs used to treat testicular cancer, as these could harm the developing foetus. I'm sure my father must have had a rather large dose while he worked his magic at bringing me into this world. It's advisable to use effective contraception during your treatment and up to a year after treatment. Condoms are advised to be used during sex within the first 48 hours after chemotherapy to protect your partner from any drugs that may be present in semen. You're obviously a better and fitter man than me if you can get it on within 2 days of treatment and must have the energy of a lion.

I had chosen to have an early night with two of the leeches that had grown attached to me, "literally" I wouldn't say I was in a bad way, but my mind was racing and I'd read War and Peace in 7 minutes, I did brail crosswords and platted the cat's hair with wire wool and live semtex. No..... I don't think the chemo really affected my state of mind. I ended up having to ask one of the leeches to leave as it was coming between me and my girl; I remember it took 13 hours to prize it off my buttock as it sucked for England.

We finally got it off by playing the banjo and teasing it with a 7lb black pudding. I'd pluck the strings and we'd strategically placed a table tennis bat at the side of the bed and placed disco lights to the side to entice it to the dance floor. It finally climbed off and down the side of the bed and switched into its night fever mode, slid on a pair of white slacks that were emblazed with the sharpest crease down the middle and a waistcoat to match. This was sucking it night fever leeches style.

It weaved and spun around the dance floor, winking at the black pudding laying by the disco lights. Courting it with spins and grooves and thrusts of its hips and groin, yes I know..... I didn't know that leeches had groins. It eventually made its move and pounced on the poor black pudding, sucking the life out of it until there was only a knob of fat left. Johnny Leech was so engrossed in his love dance that as soon as he realised he'd devoured his conquest he was looking around in disbelief and felt a sudden splurge of guilt at the pudding he'd loved and lost. He was last seen climbing out of our letter box with a suitcase, made out of a match box and hairpin. He was spotted days later stuck to the butcher's shop window, pining for black pudding to be put on special offer.

If you have any questions about your treatment don't be afraid to ask your doctor or nurse. It helped me to make a list of questions before going to appointments. And again I took my partner, but a close friend or a relative is also a good idea.

The Affects of Testicular Cancer On Sex Life and Fertility

One of the most common questions asked by men before treatment for testicular cancer is whether their sex life will be affected.

The important thing to remember is that the removal of one testicle will not affect your sexual performance or your ability to father children. If the other testicle is healthy you will also gain more living space in your boxes or Y fronts, so always think of the positive.

The remaining healthy testicle will produce more testosterone and sperm to make up for the removal of the affected testicle. You may have to have a meeting with the remaining testicle to work out shift patterns, now it's working alone, don't let it pull the wool over your eyes. If it asks for double time, for the extra work it has to put in, try and come to some compromise, we agreed no weekend work and time and a half, so everyone was happy. Also take time at least once a week to sit in a quiet spot in the house and talk to your testicle. I started sitting in the window with my head in my boxer shorts and we'd discuss the weather, football and current affairs. I was arrested twice after the neighbours complained, but it strengthened the relationship between man and ball. I caught him one day looking at a photo of his old mate and reassured him he was in a better place and not to worry. I held him in the palm of my hand and recited a Wordsworth poem, it helped .Next day I had a burning sensation in my groin, he'd remembered an argument they'd had years ago and burned the photo, he had no regard for my safety so I refused to play with him for a few days.

You're Feelings

Most people feel overwhelmed when they are told they have cancer, even with a high chance of a cure, like it can be with testicular cancer. I was on an emotional rollercoaster as different emotions surfaced. This can cause confusion and frequent mood changes. People feel different things and their reactions might not be the same as the next person, there is no right or wrong way to feel. The emotions that come to the surface are part of the process that many people go through in trying to come to terms with their illness. Partners, family members and friends often experience similar feelings and frequently need as much support and guidance in coping .At times I chose to push people away and deal with it on my own, then the next minute I would bring it up in conversation down the pub. I'd say I didn't really want to talk about it with my partner and be ignorant to the fact that she too was also frightened and may want to talk about it. Shock, disbelief and denial are the words that spring to mind.

I thought I would never be the same again, I was a lesser man! "How would my peers now see me"? Would I be able to sustain a relationship with a testicle missing? I thought I was losing part of my sexual identify and this had an immediate affect on my sexual relationship. My girlfriend would come home early from work and find me in bed with the hoover, but she never complained about bed bugs. I needed time alone and time to talk to her, she needed time too. When we talked it helped.

Uncertainty

I was unsure about the future and what it held for me. Was I still a man and what do I now need to do? The word "Cancer" frightened me. It's a word surrounded by fear. One of the greatest fears I expressed at the time of diagnosis was "Am I going to die?"

Many cancers today are curable if caught early enough. When a cancer is not completely curable, modern treatments often mean that the disease can be controlled for years and many patients can live an almost normal life.

I was anxious about the treatment I was to undergo and realised that I needed to ask questions. If your affected write a list of what you want to find out, and never ever be afraid to ask. There are no silly questions.

Anger

I was angry for a time, and confused at what I was actually angry about. I'd sit on my own feeling sorry for myself and want to run as far away from the whole business as possible. Where was I running? There was nowhere to run anyway. The battle was in my head and heart, I'd go on long walks, thinking why has this happened and would I ever be able to enjoy the normal things in life. The flowers, the sea, football - would I be able to laugh freely again with no shadow over me. It was a deeply humbling time for me and for my loved ones.

Blame

I wanted to blame everything, everyone, the tight jeans in the 1980s I wore, the meals my girlfriend cooked me, my over enthusiastic masturbating as a teenager. Was it the size 8-10 year old Y fronts I wore as a 17 year old? Was it the smoke in pubs I put myself in at the time. I would quietly sit and question everything I had done in the past and look for a reason why I had cancer. I would resent people who were healthy or who I thought were fine and the fact that I had to deal with this untimely illness while they were getting on with their normal lives. Thankfully these thoughts pass and there is the realisation that there is no one to blame, its no ones fault. It is not some kind of punishment for wearing my mums dress as a 4 year old.....it is just life. People are touched by these things every day.

In time I found it was great to talk to people about it, and I confided in friends and family and to be honest anyone that would listen.

The Symptoms of Testicular Cancer

The most common symptom is swelling in one part of the testicle. This is usually painless, but some men, me included can notice an ache, in their lower abdomen or in the affected testicle. There maybe also feelings of "heaviness" in the scrotum. In a few cases the testicle can suddenly become swollen and very tender.

When examined, a healthy testicle feels round, soft and smooth.

The epidiydmis can be felt behind it as a separate structure. Cysts and benign swellings in the peidiydiuis are quite common and are usually harmless. Lumps in the body of the testes itself may be benign but can be cancer.

If you have any swellings then go to the doctors. If I'm in your town I will give you a lift myself.

A few men may find that their first symptoms (such as backache, stomach ache) are caused by the spread of the cancer cells to other parts of the body. Rarely, tender nipples may be caused by hormonal changes. Come to think of it "Tender Nipples" was the name of the wrestler that used to grapple with my old boss. Most of these symptoms are usually harmless and it's likely to be due to conditions other than cancer.

Examine yourself about once a month, after a warm bath or shower, when the scrotam skin is relaxed. Have some quality one time with your testicles and get to know them again. It can be lonely place in a pair of Y fronts or boxes or scrunched up in a bright purple thong waiting for action.

If you have swelling in your testicles, it's important to get your GP to examine you. If I hadn't I may not have had a beautiful son.

Causes of Testicular Cancer

The causes of testicular cancer are not yet fully understood. However, research has identified a number of factors which may increase your chances of developing the condition. Some of these risk factors are outlined below.

Undescended Testicles

The medical name for undescended testicles is cryptorchidism. When male babies grow in the womb, their testicles develop inside their abdomen. The testicles then normally move down into the scrotum when the baby is born, or during their first year of life. However, for some children, the testicles fail to descend into the scrotum. Surgery is normally required to move the testicles down. If your testicles require surgery because they do not descend, it may increase the risk of you developing testicular cancer. One study found that if surgery is performed before the child is 13 years of age, their risk of testicular cancer is approximately double than that of the rest of the population. However, if the operation is carried out after the boy is 13 years of age, or older, the risk of developing testicular cancer is five times greater than that of the rest of the population.

Age and Race

Unlike most other cancers, testicular cancer is more common in young and middle-aged men, than in older, or elderly, men. It most commonly affects men who are between 20-44 years of age, with 90% of testicular cancer cases affecting men who are under the age of age 55. Testicular cancer is also more common in white men, compared with other racial groups. It is also more common in northern and western Europe than in any other part of the world.

Close Family Member

If a close family member has had testicular cancer, such as your father, or brother, it may increase your risk of developing the condition. It is thought that approximately 1 in 5 cases of testicular cancer are the result of an inherited faulty gene.

Types of Testicular Cancer

There are two main types of testicular cancer:

Seminoma & non-Seminoma

The terms Seminoma and non-Seminoma refer to the type of cell that makes up the cancerous tumour. Seminoma testicular cancers only contain Seminoma cells. Non-Seminomas may contain a variety of different cancer cells. However, both types of testicular cancer are treated in a similar way. Testicular cancer is also a type of germ cell cancer. A germ cell cancer is one that starts in the cells that are used to make sperm or eggs (ovarian cancer is another type of germ cell cancer).

Sperm Storage Before Treatment For Testicular Cancer

If your sperm is suitable and you would like to store some for the future, you will need to produce a number of sperm samples over a period of time. These can be frozen and stored for some time by the hospital, when you want to father a child, your sperm can be thawed and used to artificially inseminate your partner. Unfortunately not every man has sperm suitable for banking. To be successfully stored it is thought that a sample must contain a certain number of active sperm cells, which would be able to fertilise a female egg. However new technology now make it possible for less active sperm to be effective. Active sperm can also be taken from the testes even when they are not in the ejaculate. Discuss this with your doctor, sperm storage before any treatment starts so that test can be done to check your sperm count. For many patients with cancer, the cancer unit will provide free sperm banking. But if the hospital has to pay for this service, it may need to charge the patient. The costs vary between hospitals.

Giving Consent to Treatment for Testicular Cancer

Before you have any treatments your doctor will explain the aims of the treatment to you. They will usually ask you to sign a form saying that you give your permission (consent) for the hospital staff to give you the treatment. No medical treatment can be given, without your consent and before you are asked to sign the form you should have been given full information about the type of treatment and extent. Advantages and disadvantages of the treatment;

- Any possible other treatments that may be available
- Any significant risks or side effects of the treatment.

If you do not understand what you are hearing, let the staff know straight away. It's not unusual for people to need repeated explanations. Again it would be a good idea to take a relative or partner or a friend with you, to help you remember the discussion fully. It's important to know how the treatment may affect you, so it's good to ask as many questions as possible. The staff are always willing to help. Remember you can always ask for more time to decide about the treatment and are free to choose not to have the treatment, whatever your decision, it needs recording in your medical notes. You don't need to give a reason for not wanting to have treatment, but it can be helpful to let the staff know your concerns so that they can give you the best advice.

Research Clinical Trials

Research into new ways of treating testicular cancer are reducing the side effects of treatment, it is going on all the time. When a new treatment is being developed, it goes through various stages of research. First it is looked at in the laboratory and sometimes tested on cancer cells in a test tube. If the treatment seems as though it might be useful in treating cancer, it is given to patients in research studies (clinical trials). These early studies are called Phase 1 trials aim to:
- Find a safe dose
- See what side effects the therapy may cause
- Identify which cancers it might be used to treat

If early studies suggest that a new treatment may be both safe and effective, further trials (Phase 2 and 3) are done to answer these questions:

- Is it better than existing treatments?
- Does it have extra benefit with existing treatments?
- How does it compare with the current best standard treatments?

You may be asked to take part in a research trial. There can be many benefits in doing this. You will be helping to improve knowledge about cancer and the development of new treatments. You will also be carefully monitored during and after the study.

It is important to be aware that some treatments that look promising at first are often later found to be not as good as existing treatments, or have side effects that outweigh any benefits. As part of research you may be asked by your doctors for permission to store some samples of your tumour or blood, so that they can be used as part of trials to find the causes of cancer.

Be Good………Check your nuts……..Laugh a lot……Help others and Help yourself !

The End

I've Only got One, but It's a BEAUTY

Lightning Source UK Ltd.
Milton Keynes UK
178295UK00001B/19/P